More Advance Praise for

Inside the Dementia Epidemic

"A remarkable, brutally honest, and beautifully written account of what it's like to take on the role of caregiver for a loved one with dementia. Martha takes us on a brave journey from at-home care to the difficult decision of choosing to have professionals care for her mother in a residential facility. There is heartbreak, joy, and incredibly useful information in this touching memoir that will help anyone facing the task of taking care of an elderly person who can no longer take care of themselves."

—**Mary Ellen Geist,** author of *Measure of the Heart: A Father's Alzheimer's, a Daughter's Return*

"With the passion of a committed daughter and the fervor of a tireless reporter, Martha Stettinius weaves a compelling story of her long journey caregiving for her demented mother with a broad exploration of the causes of dementia, means of treating it, and hopes for preventing it. Her greatest gift to readers is that of optimism—that caregiving can deepen love, that dementia can be fought, and that families can be strengthened. Her book is appealing, enlightening, inspiring."

—**Barry J. Jacobs, Psy.D.,** author of *The Emotional Survival Guide for Caregivers—Looking After Yourself and Your Family While Helping an Aging Parent*

"*Inside the Dementia Epidemic* is special, because it combines a very personal story about how a daughter is affected by her mother's illness with a broader perspective on Alzheimer's disease and other dementias. This book is a guide for everyone hit by Alzheimer's and dementia, and it reads very well."

—**Marc Wortmann,** Executive Director, Alzheimer's Disease International

"Many writers have reflected on the experience of being a son or daughter of a person living with dementia, but until I read *Inside the Dementia Epidemic* I had not found one that pulled off the remarkable feat of helping the reader understand and actually feel the journey of both parent and child. This remarkable book is invaluable precisely because it offers us a deeply honest account of both perspectives."

—**Jude Thomas**, Care Partner, and Co-Founder of The Eden Alternative

"Martha Stettinius has a wonderful style of writing that ignites vivid images. Her first-person style conveys well the family experience with a loved one with dementia: at turns confusing, challenging, heartbreaking, and joyful. Other families going through similar challenges will gain from the stories and the knowledge Martha collects along the way."

— **Sharon K. Brothers, MSW**, Senior Vice President, Caregiver Village, and CEO, Institute for Professional Care Education

"A wonderful, heartfelt diary of what it feels like to be a family member of someone with an irreversible dementia. *Inside the Dementia Epidemic* is valuable not only for family members who sometimes feel as if they are alone in this journey, but also for healthcare professionals who need to understand the impact this disease has on families. Martha writes not only from the heart (how it feels) but from her head (what she would have done and asked over the years, had she known then what she knows now), and that is the strength of this book."

—**Joyce Simard, MSW**, Adjunct Associate Professor, University of Western Sydney, Australia; geriatric consultant and author, *The End-of-Life Namaste Care Program for People with Dementia*

"Readers who are challenged with caring for a loved one suffering from dementia will find much to guide them in this chronicle of a daughter's journey to help her mother through the several stages of this dreadful disease. A moving and insightful work."

—**Claire Berman**, author of *Caring for Yourself While Caring for Your Aging Parents: How to Help, How to Survive*

"A thoughtful and beautifully written book. Martha Stettinius is honest in recording not just the practical difficulties she encounters as she navigates a path through the complex and often illogical world of dementia care services, but also the emotional journey she makes. Martha generously shares the practical, financial, and medical information she has learned, and the emotional insights she has gleaned.

"This book will help you appreciate that you are not alone, but part of a wider community of people who have all been caught up in the 'dementia epidemic.'"

—**Lucy Whitman**, editor of *Telling Tales About Dementia: Experiences of Caring*

"An honest, emotionally-charged, and thought-provoking account and life story of the author's mother and the dementia journey. Many moments in the book literally took my breath away and made me really think about the dementia journey and the impact this diagnosis has not only on the person but the family who loves and cares for them."

—**Sandra Stimson, CALA, ADC, CDP, CDCM, AC-BC**
Founder and Executive Director, National
Council of Certified Dementia Practitioners

"Dementia is an all-consuming and intimate disease, the effects of which linger long after the death of the loved one. Readers will not only find Martha Stettinius's memoir consoling, they will gain the invaluable advantage of hindsight on things she would do differently if she had to do it all over again."

—**Joy Loverde**, author of *The Complete Eldercare Planner, Revised and Updated Edition: Where to Start, Which Questions to Ask, and How to Find Help*

"I've personally found inspiration and deep wisdom in the story Martha tells. She offers the reader—whether we're now a caregiver, have been one, or possibly will be in the future—an understanding of the challenges and changes that can face the family caregiver. Her beautiful and honest tale deserves our deepest gratitude."

—**Connie Goldman**, speaker and author of *The Gifts of Caregiving—Stories of Hardship, Hope and Healing*

"Martha shares from her heart her struggles to find peace for both herself and her mother as they navigate through the challenges of Alzheimer's disease. *Inside the Dementia Epidemic* is an excellent, eye-opening account of what Alzheimer's caregivers go through."

—**Nataly Rubinstein, MSW, LCSW, C-ASWCM**, Alzheimer's Care Consultants, Inc., and author of *Alzheimer's Disease and Other Dementias: The Caregiver's Complete Survival Guide*

"*Inside the Dementia Epidemic* joins a growing body of tales in books and the popular press that describe the poignant, trying experience of devoted family members dealing with the implications of dementia. This story captures well the personal cost of care as a daughter helps her mother through the various levels of the disease and treatment modalities. It reminds us of the terrible toll this disease takes on everyone who comes in contact with it. We have no simple fixes—no medications, no care systems that can make the consequences easier to bear.

"People facing this challenge can read this book to find solace that they are not alone, their frustrations are not of their own making, and no one has the easy answers."

—**Robert L. Kane, MD,** Minnesota Chair in Long-term Care and Aging, University of Minnesota School of Public Health, and author of *It Shouldn't Be This Way: The Failure of Long-term Care* and *The Good Caregiver*

"*Inside the Dementia Epidemic* is much more than a traditional memoir. Martha lets the reader join her personal caregiver's journey with beautifully executed phrasing, skillful storytelling, and hardcore facts. A fascinating and informative read that not only educates, but touches the heart."

—**Carol Bradley Bursack,** Founder and Owner, Minding Our Elders, and author of *Minding Our Elders: Caregivers Share Their Personal Stories*

"Martha Stettinius shares many of the great lessons of 'care partnering' for someone with dementia—not just how to navigate the system, but how to enjoy her time with her mother. Her reflections throughout the book about what she has learned will help others realize early on that they should question their interactions and seek out the best interventions."

—**Kerry Mills,** President, Engaging Alzheimer's

"As a nurse, dementia consultant, and daughter of a parent with dementia, I can tell you without hesitation to read *Inside the Dementia Epidemic* if you have a loved one with dementia in your life. Martha's insights will help you understand why you feel as you do, and why you shouldn't beat yourself up about it. She includes a wealth of information about the many issues families face. You will be glad you found this book to help guide you."

—**Cindy Keith, RN, BS,** Certified Dementia Practitioner, author of *Love, Laughter, and Mayhem —Caregiver Survival Manual for Living with a Person with Dementia,* and owner of M.I.N.D. in Memory Care

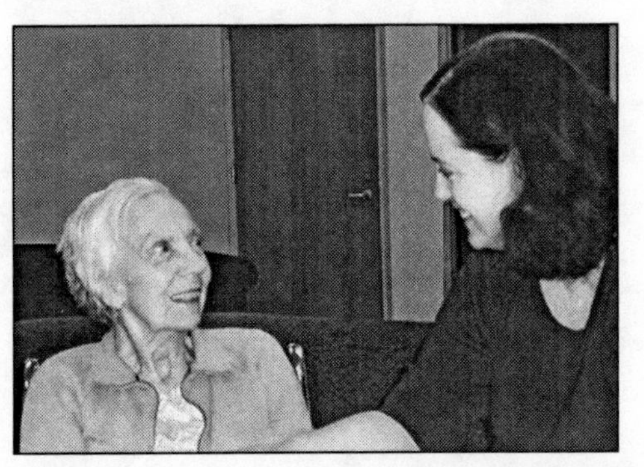

My mother, Judy, and me at her nursing home in the spring of 2012.

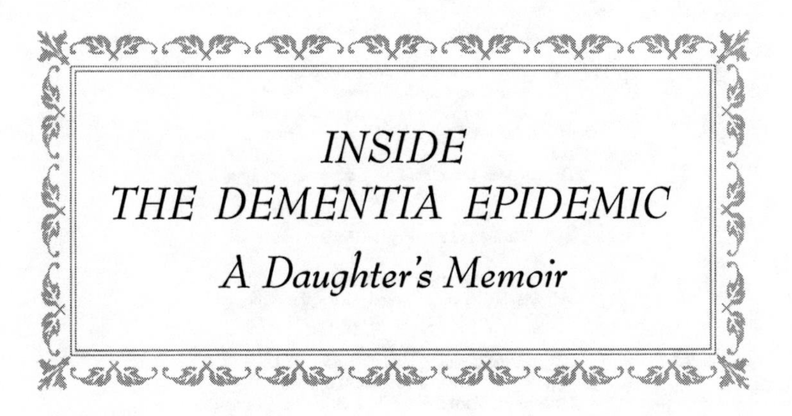

INSIDE THE DEMENTIA EPIDEMIC

A Daughter's Memoir

Martha Stettinius

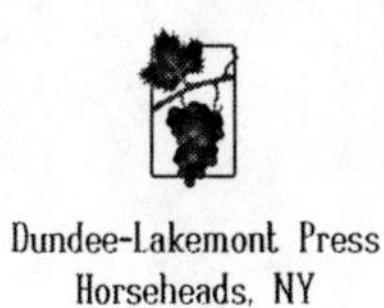

Dundee-Lakemont Press
Horseheads, NY

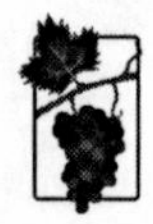

DUNDEE-LAKEMONT PRESS
110 N Main St
HORSEHEADS, NY 14845

First Dundee-Lakemont Press trade paperback edition
September 2012

Publisher's Cataloging-in-Publication data

Stettinius, Martha.
Inside the dementia epidemic : a daughter's memoir /
by Martha Stettinius.
p. cm.
Includes bibliographical references and index.
ISBN 978-0-9849326-0-3 (pbk.)
1. Stettinius, Martha —Family. 2. Dementia —Patients
—Family relationships. 3. Dementia —Patients
—Home Care. 4. Mothers and daughters —United States.
5. Caregivers —Biography. I. Title.
RC521 .S745 2012 362.196/83 --dc23
2012936984
Printed in the United States of America
10 9 8 7 6 5 4 3 2 1

Cover by Susan Koski Zucker
Book design by Heather McCarty
Author photo by Sheryl Sinkow

For information regarding special discounts for bulk
purchases, please contact Dundee-Lakemont Press at
info@dundee-lakemontpress.com

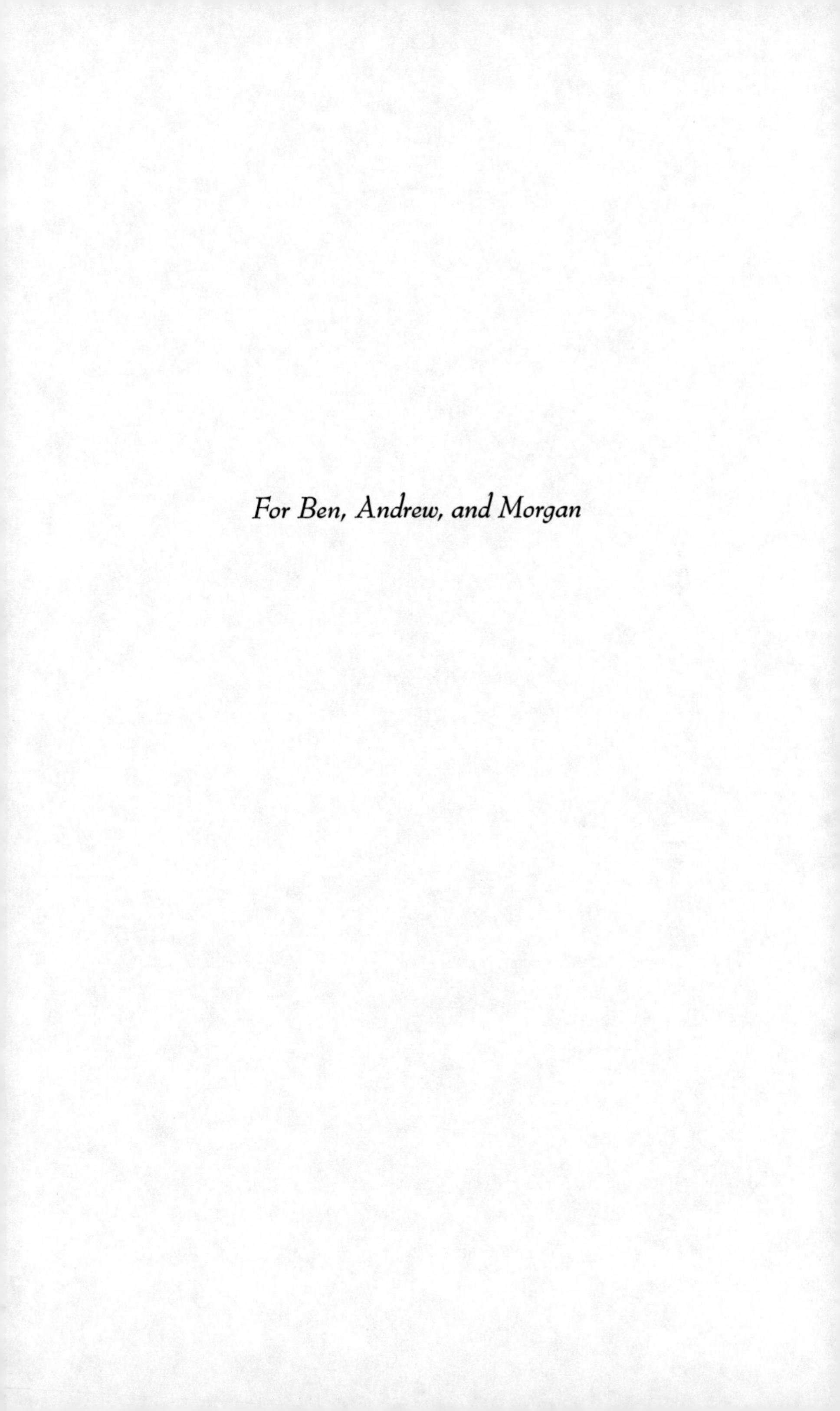

For Ben, Andrew, and Morgan

Care-partners—family, friends, professionals and governments—should actively seek to understand the person's needs, take full account of existing capabilities, and adjust care levels according to those needs. Listen to us as we try to express these needs and abilities. That way we can dance in celebration together and embrace our shared future.

— CHRISTINE BRYDEN, *Dancing with Dementia: My Story of Living Positively with Dementia*

Contents

Author's Note

This is a true story. To ensure privacy I have changed the names and identifying characteristics of the places and people I mention, with the exception of myself, my mother, and other members of my family. To ensure the accuracy of my scenes, I kept a journal and recorded all the details and conversations shortly after they took place.

I have striven at all times to be honest, but also fair and compassionate. And although I am not a professional in dementia care—I'm a daughter and a family caregiver—my research has been thorough, and portions of my text have been reviewed by experts in dementia.

—M.S., July 2012

INSIDE THE DEMENTIA EPIDEMIC:
A Daughter's Memoir

Preface

For seven years I have coped with my mother's dementia. I have cared for her at home, in assisted living, a rehab center, a specialized "memory care" facility, and the dreaded nursing home.

What do we face next?

In my question lies hope. Hope not just for my mother, Judy, but for me, and for you.

The journey I have taken with my mother has alerted me to the latest scientific findings about dementia. Although the facts are frightening, they are our only hope if we wish to emerge with our minds intact from what is now a fast-growing epidemic.

The shocking wake-up call is that this epidemic will also overtake those of us in middle age, unless we can somehow prevent or treat it.

One in eight people over age sixty-five in the United States has Alzheimer's disease, and nearly fifty percent over age eighty-five. In 2012, an estimated 5.4 million people in the United States will have Alzheimer's disease. As people continue to live longer, and the baby boomers grow older, the number of people with dementia will explode. The 35.6 million with dementia worldwide in 2010 is expected to double by 2030 to 65.7 million, and then nearly double again by 2050 to 115.4 million.

Even if we do not get the disease, or if we get it late in life, we are likely to become a family caregiver for someone with dementia. In the United States in 2011, over 15 million family caregivers provided 17.4 billion hours of unpaid care to family members and friends with Alzheimer's disease and other dementias. This unpaid care was estimated to be worth $210.5 billion, more than the total for federal and state Medicare and Medicaid spending for Alzheimer's care. Family caregivers often sacrifice their own health and finances to provide that care. A third of family caregivers report feeling depressed, and sixty percent feel extreme stress.

Dementia is not only Alzheimer's (the most common, at sixty to eighty percent), but a Pandora's Box diagnosis that includes over one hundred conditions. Familial Alzheimer's—also called "early-onset" dementia—occurs before the age of sixty, and represents 5-7 percent of Alzheimer's cases. "Mixed dementia"—Alzheimer's plus another type of dementia—has been shown in autopsies to occur in up to 45 percent of people with dementia. Vascular dementia alone, of which there are several forms, accounts for up to 20 percent of dementias.

This book is not a lament, however; it is a guide, and, I hope, a means to soften the blow upon all of us. In the course of my own experience, I discovered what could have been done earlier to help my mother, and what can be done *now* to help us all: Startling scientific findings show that certain changes in diet and exercise—even changes in eye care and sleep patterns—may decrease the risk of developing these diseases. If we are to survive the "silver tsunami," which will overwhelm half the population in the not-too-distant future, we must join the worldwide movement demanding more dementia research. Alzheimer's disease is the fifth-leading cause of death in the United States for those age 65 and older, but the only one in the top ten without a means of prevention, a way to slow its progression for more than a few years, or a cure.

Even if by luck or a preventive lifestyle we don't succumb to dementia, each of us will pay for its treatment. In the United States in 2012, Medicare, Medicaid and out-of-pocket expenditures for Alzheimer's and other dementia care total $200 billion. By 2050, the projected cost will reach $1.1 trillion. William Thies, Ph.D., the Alzheimer's Association's Chief Medical and Scientific Officer, says that "the overwhelming number of people whose lives will be altered by Alzheimer's disease and dementia, combined with the staggering burden on families and nations, make Alzheimer's the defining disease of this generation."

Remember those words as you read this book:

"The defining disease of this generation."

The good news is that it is not too late to save yourself, and to learn how to best support your relatives if they already suffer.

By sharing my journey of discovery, as well as the resources I acquired during the past seven years, I hope to help you cope with your afflicted family members and friends. What I've learned also might help you save your own sanity.

Over the past few years I've inhaled all of the memoirs I could find about dementia caregiving, but most of these memoirs by adult children caring for a parent with dementia either treat the elder as hapless and amusing, which I find disrespectful, or they focus on the extreme stress and craziness of caregiving at home with little support. Few of these caregivers have written scenes in multiple care settings, as I have; few describe how they found adequate assistance; and few offer hope that the caregiving journey can be anything other than a crushing self-sacrifice. They describe dementia itself as a tragic wasting away and a long, painful goodbye—indeed, as the complete erasure of the person who once was. What I have experienced and felt with Mom is different, and I want to share our story.

Related essays on dementia research, dementia risk factors, and planning for long-term care can be found in the appendices.

I have navigated the maze of choices inherent in dementia care, and I can now offer my journey as a guide. With enough support from others, caregiving need not mean a life of constant exhaustion and loss. These years can be both manageable and meaningful—not a "long good-bye" as it's often described, but a "long hello."

Part I

HOME CARE

Judy

A minor car mishap signals the end of what had been my former relationship with my mother, and the beginning of my major involvement in her care.

It is a February day in 2005, crisp after a fresh snow. I am following my mother's car from her cottage on a lake to her doctor's office in the small town nearby. I hadn't planned to follow my mother for safety reasons, only as a routine need to have two cars for our separate plans later in the day.

Although she's driven through this town for twenty-five years, Mom loses her way and misses the block by the doctor's office. When she finally pulls over to the side of the road, her car starts to slip into a ditch.

This isn't the first time I've seen my mother do this. When I was fourteen, my mother and I had been at the cottage alone one weekend, and she had been drinking as usual. As we headed back to our house two hours away, Mom turned twenty feet too early at the main road and drove the car five feet down into a ditch. She had to call a tow truck and explain to strangers how, on a clear, sunny evening, she ended up in the ditch.

But on this snowy day, instead of reversing or summoning help, my mother continues to accelerate forward until she is wedged downward at so steep an angle that the front end of her Honda Accord is buried in the snow and the rear end of the car sticks up three feet in the air. I pull my mother from the driver's seat and call another tow truck.

This drama symbolized the facts: At seventy-two, my mother was beginning to fall into a great white opacity. It was up to me to save her. What would have happened to her if I had not followed her car? The image of my mother—trapped, pointed downward into nothingness—haunts me, still.

Judy is not just a thin, white-haired woman whose sky-blue eyes are eerily bright. Judy is a complicated, unusual person in her own right. Thirty years ago, twice divorced, Mom sold our home as soon as I left for college and moved to our family's vacation house—a two-story cottage on Silver Lake in rural New York. Then forty-nine years old, she cut her ties with ordinary life—her teaching job, commuting, and suburban settings. Without the usual obligations, my mother entered the world of her weekends and summer holidays. Judy set herself free, in a way many people wish to do, but few dare.

Now, whenever I have to move my mother from one facility to the next, following the stages of her deterioration, I carry the framed photograph that, in my mind, shows the "real Judy"—Judy at her best.

In this picture, you see a vital fifty-four-year-old woman, brunette, tanned brown, in a light-blue canoe, her dog beside her. This was the year of my mother's great solo expedition around her beloved Silver Lake, thirty-three miles on each side. She carried a tent, sleeping bag, dried food, water, a Bunsen burner, a journal, and her miniature Schnauzer.

Her plan was to interview the lake people, camp on the shores, and collect an oral history for a comprehensive chronicle of the mysterious, six-hundred-foot-deep lake famous for its "Guns of Silver," the underwater booms that echo like explosions through the valleys and vineyards. The source of the thunder may be natural gas escaping from pockets in the bedrock beneath the lake. (That legend may now be a liability. Even as I write, there are news reports that my mother's lake is threatened by the prospect of gas drilling along its shores that would destroy the ecological balance. As Judy is endangered, so is the place she loved.)

The twenty-five years my mother spent living alone in that remote lake house represented the most successful, idiosyncratic stretch in her life. Mom called herself "Woodswoman," inspired by Anne LaBastille's book about living alone in the Adirondack Mountains. Mom took pride in chopping and stacking her own wood for the fireplace, and loved to be outside whenever she could, working in the yard. She enjoyed the quiet off-season when she had the expanse of lake nearly all to herself. She said, "a life lived indoors is no life at all."

Judy planned to live the rest of her life at the cottage. She loved the early morning sun rising wide and roseate over cliffs on the opposite shore, the waves changing direction without warning from north to south and south to north. Because of its depth, and its constant turning over from bottom to top, the lake freezes only once in a hundred years. From her desk facing the picture windows, Mom could see the winter waves fifty feet away crash fierce and white-tipped into the railroad-tie breakwall.

It is one of the cruel ironies of dementia that this very beautiful, natural lifestyle, which gave her such pleasure, may have hastened my mother's decline. As you will see in the appendices, new findings indicate that the brain must be stimulated; we must continually challenge our minds to learn new skills, and to participate in a variety of social and cultural events. Not only was Mom's solitary life dangerous, but her deterioration was well advanced before anyone knew.

Mom first showed signs of vascular dementia (also called "multi-infarct dementia") from small strokes at age sixty-five. She is now, at age seventy-nine in 2012, in the last stage of "mixed dementia"—in her case, most likely a combination of Alzheimer's disease and vascular dementia.

I became my mother's sole family caregiver at the age of forty, a job I never expected, and at first resisted. Because of our complex history together, I denied as long as I could that she needed help. My relationship with my mother had gone through its own stages and upheavals. Through the years I have been angry with her, estranged from her, and devoted to her.

The day after she drove herself into that first ditch, my mother put herself into treatment for alcoholism. For the rest of her life, she stayed sober but continued to struggle with depression, anxiety, and obsessive-compulsive personality disorder. I left home at sixteen, and, for many years, had a long-distance relationship with her. Visits were strained. (I remember the dramas—the night I fled, pregnant, with my stunned, young husband, when my mother ordered us to leave the cottage into a cold, black rain.) In different periods in our lives, we tried to overcome the tensions between us, aided by counseling and 12-step programs, but I kept my distance.

Then, the slide into the snow ditch, and everything changed. I slid as well, blind and ignorant, into the dementia epidemic. I had no reason to know about the intricacies of the different settings for dementia care, let alone how to pay for them. As a matter of fact, I began writing this book because I felt guilty about each decision I had made on my mother's behalf. I needed to figure out if my choices were sound or selfish. I knew no one else at age forty balancing the care of children and a parent, and feared that, with caregiving on top of work and family, I would lose myself. I also questioned the idea, so prevalent today, that to "age in place," to receive care at home, is inherently better for elders than care in a facility.

I would learn that, for many of us, becoming a caregiver for one's parent is a midlife coming-of-age. I now emerge from the upheaval of this transition more confident, willing to ask for help, attuned to my own needs, and appreciative of the simple gifts of life.

The Decision

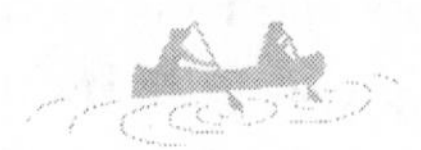

A month before my mother drove into the ditch across from her doctor's office, she had called him in a panic. She couldn't remember if she'd recorded a certain check. Dr. Gavin and I both knew how meticulous she was with her checkbook. This incident upset her so much that she called me, too, which was also unlike her.

On the phone she told me that the previous night she had lost her bearing outside in the dark and almost stepped off a cliff. "And two weeks before that," she'd said, "I fell on my way down the hill from the car. I wasn't hurt, but I'm scared. What if I fall again, Martha? What if get confused again and walk off that cliff?" She confessed her concerns all at once, as if she could no longer hide them from me.

It was clear my mother could no longer live alone at the cottage. It was simply too dangerous.

What would be the alternative? Should I start commuting to care for her on a regular basis? I lived almost two hours away, round-trip. I worked. I had two young children. If Mom continued to live at the cottage, she would need someone to shop, cook all her meals for her, and clean. The cottage was five miles from the nearest town, which was too small to offer transportation services for the elderly, and few neighbors lived on the lake in the off-season to help drive her to appointments.

I thought of the access road down the cliff to the cottages. It was blasted perhaps a hundred years ago, with the narrow passage hugging the cliff at a forty-five-degree angle, and a hairpin curve halfway down the steep descent. Once in a while, the only other year-round neighbor plowed the road with his four-wheel-drive; but even then, most cars couldn't make it up and down the road without threatening to slip sideways off the cliff. My mother had to park her car on a precipice five hundred feet up the road, and clamber up and down with her packages.

How had my mother managed this? Like a Nordic explorer, she wore ice cleats on her boots for traction and held a ski pole in her hand for balance. She baby-stepped up the hill to her car, then carried her groceries and library books back down in a red backpack. When she was younger, she pulled an improvised sled, a blue, plastic barrel cut in half with a rope attached.

For her to continue to travel to and from her cottage would tempt a deadly accident. What could I do?

I discarded the idea of commuting to drive her to and fro, or hiring aides to do so. Even at that starting point, I could see the potential problems with weather and no-show aides.

Maybe she could move in with me, my husband Ben, and our children? I assumed that it would be easier for me, less stressful, if she lived in our home where I could include her in our meals, help plan her activities, and attend to her other needs without driving. I imagined that having my mother live with us would be the easiest way for me to help her.

My family lives in an unusual, planned community, a development of more than thirty families on a large parcel of mostly open land. I imagined that, if my mother needed more company than I could give her, all I would need to do would be to walk across the gravel path that connects the houses and knock on a door, call someone, or send an email on the community's listserv.

I pictured Mom smiling and serene as she sits with a new friend at a concert at one of the three universities in town; joining us three nights a week for community meals; watching neighbors of all ages weave the cloth ribbons of our Maypole in the spring. I assumed that my role would be peripheral. Our community would give Mom the stimulation she needs to rejoin the pulse of life.

Most important, though, I wanted to protect my mother—keep her from falling or starving. She looked skeletal, and I wanted to feed her. In my home, I could tuck her under my wing as I would my children; I could send her out into the world but watch her.

I talked to Ben about her living with us. He has not had warm feelings for my mother since that night, early in our marriage, when she kicked us out of the cottage in a rage. Ben agreed to invite my mother into our home only because it was important to me.

I called Mom to tell her that it was too dangerous for her to stay at the cottage any longer, that she could live with us. I was sure she would balk. To my surprise, she seemed relieved.

She said, "You're right, honey," her voice small and far away. "I don't think I can do this anymore."

When we finally do reach Dr. Gavin's office that February morning, I report the incident of the snow ditch. Mom is quite fond of the elderly Dr. Gavin, her "small town doctor," as she calls him, and has been going to him since she moved into the cottage.

He reads aloud what he records in my mother's chart: "Judy's daughter is uncertain at this time whether or not her mother should be driving."

Turning to Mom, he says, "I believe you may have had a very small stroke, Judy."

"I have?" Mom looks startled.

"Yes, I believe so. A very small stroke, too small to detect, but one that has affected your memory." He pauses. "You and I have both noticed some small changes in your memory, haven't we?"

"Yes, I must say I've noticed," Mom says. "It's very upsetting." She frowns but continues to study the doctor's face.

Dr. Gavin asks, "Judy, could you tell me what you had for breakfast this morning?"

"I usually have ice water."

"And what did you have for lunch?"

"Crackers, I guess. I haven't been that hungry."

"Did you know that you've lost fifteen pounds this past year? You're down to 118."

"No, I had no idea."

She smiles and flutters a laugh, but I feel something chill crack. *Ice water*. She's doing even worse than I thought.

I tell Dr. Gavin that I've invited my mother to live with me.

The muscles in his face relax. Slowly, as if choosing each word carefully, he says, "I think it would be...good...for you, Judy, to be with your daughter."

"Yes, I think so, too." My mother trusts her doctor. I know she trusts me, too, but Dr. Gavin's opinion means just a bit more to her.

As I stride back down the hall with Mom at my side, I smile too much at the nurse and the assistants. I leave confident in my new role but puzzled by the doctor's reserve and his sad eyes.

A New Beginning

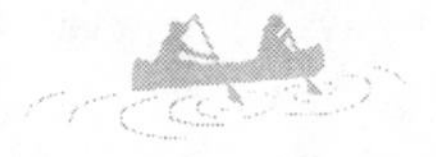

With the benefit of hindsight, I can see that my mother's behavior over the past fifteen years fit into the stages of Alzheimer's disease. Alarms were sounding but I knew too little to take advantage of what medication exists to relieve the symptoms. Had I known the stages of Alzheimer's, I might have been able to help my mother earlier, and in that way, helped myself as well. Knowing what I do now, I realize that, the day she slid her car into the snow ditch, my mother was already in Stage Four.

I outline the stages on the following pages, in order that you may be better informed than I was.

Dementia usually progresses so slowly that, as family members and friends, we can deny or rationalize for many years the changes we see in our loved ones. If they are over age eighty when diagnosed, they might live as little as three to four years, but if they are younger when diagnosed, they can live with the disease for up to twenty years. It's also difficult to label a person's behavior, as

The Alzheimer's Association describes 7 Stages of Alzheimer's Disease:

Stage 1: Normal functioning. The person's doctor, family and friends cannot detect a problem.

Stage 2: Very mild cognitive decline, which may be normal aging or early dementia. The person may forget words or where to find objects. No symptoms can be detected by a doctor, family or friends.

Stage 3: Mild cognitive decline. Sometimes Alzheimer's can be diagnosed at this stage. A doctor, family or friends may notice problems with memory or concentration. The person may:

- Have noticeable problems coming up with the right word or name
- Have trouble remembering names when introduced to new people
- Have noticeably greater difficulty performing tasks in social or work settings
- Forget material they have just read
- Lose or misplace a valuable object
- Have increasing trouble with planning or organizing

Stage 4: Moderate cognitive decline. Mild or early-stage Alzheimer's disease. A cognitive assessment by a doctor should be able to detect this stage. The person may:

- Forget recent events
- Experience an impaired ability to perform challenging mental arithmetic—for example, counting backward from 100 by 7's
- Experience greater difficulty performing complex

tasks, such as planning dinner for guests, paying bills or managing finances

Experience forgetfulness about their own personal history

Become moody or withdrawn, especially in socially or mentally challenging situations

Stage 5: Moderately severe cognitive decline. Moderate or mid-stage Alzheimer's disease. Problems with memory, cognitive tasks, or judgment are noticeable, and the person needs help with daily activities such as cooking, cleaning and paying bills. The person may:

Be unable to recall their own address or telephone number or the high school or college from which they graduated

Become confused about where they are or what day it is

Have trouble with less challenging mental arithmetic, such as counting backward from 40 by subtracting 4's or from 20 by 2's

Need help choosing proper clothing for the season or the occasion

Still remember significant details about themselves and their family

Still require no assistance with eating or using the toilet

Stage 6: Severe cognitive decline. Moderately severe or mid-stage Alzheimer's disease. The person may:

Lose awareness of recent experiences as well as of their surroundings

Remember their own name but have difficulty with their personal history

Distinguish familiar and unfamiliar faces but have trouble

remembering the name of a spouse or caregiver

Need help dressing properly and may, without supervision, make mistakes such as putting pajamas over daytime clothes or shoes on the wrong feet

Experience major changes in sleep patterns—sleeping during the day and becoming restless at night

Need help handling details of toileting (for example, flushing the toilet, wiping or disposing of tissue properly)

Have increasingly frequent trouble controlling their bladder or bowels

Experience major personality and behavioral changes, including suspiciousness and delusions (such as believing that their caregiver is an impostor) or compulsive, repetitive behavior like hand-wringing or tissue shredding

Tend to wander or become lost

Stage 7: Very severe cognitive decline. Severe or late-stage Alzheimer's disease. This stage may last from several weeks to several years. The person may:

Lose the ability to respond to their environment, to carry on a conversation and, eventually, to control movement. They may still say words or phrases.

Need help with much of their daily personal care, including eating or using the toilet.

Need assistance walking, then cannot walk at all.

Lose the ability to smile, to sit without support and to hold their heads up. Reflexes become abnormal. Muscles grow rigid. Swallowing becomes impaired.

Death often occurs from pneumonia from aspirated food.

In May of 2011 an international workgroup of more than forty top Alzheimer's researchers will recommend that Alzheimer's disease be broken down into three wider stages:

The preclinical stage
"Mild cognitive impairment (MCI) due to Alzheimer's disease," and
"Dementia due to Alzheimer's disease."

With mild cognitive impairment, problems with memory and cognitive ability are noticeable, but don't affect the person's ability to take care of themselves from day to day. Not everyone who has mild cognitive impairment will develop Alzheimer's disease. In the third stage, "dementia due to Alzheimer's disease," independence in day-to-day function becomes difficult, then impossible.

the stages often overlap from year to year, and may even seem to change from day to day or hour to hour.

After the visit with Dr. Gavin, I experience the mood and decision reversals that further reveal my mother's instability. Mom calls me to tell me that she cried and cried all morning.

"Why are you making me move in with you?" she asks. She says she called her neighbor Susan who told her, "You shouldn't need help if you can still write your own checks."

I feel myself beginning to shake. This neighbor has managed to undermine all my tentative progress with Mom. Yes, she can write checks, but she forgets why she's writing them, how much they're for, and how to enter them in her check register. Mom cannot remember why she was excited to move in with us, and I have to explain it all for the twentieth time. I remind her of the fall, the disorientation on the dark road, the weight loss.

Mom laughs—a nervous laugh—on the other end of the phone. "I thought I had to move because I have a few cobwebs in the house."

"No, it's much worse than that, Mom. You seem"—I search for the right word; I want her to know how serious this is—"disconnected...from all of the trash around you."

Months earlier, I had been shocked by my discoveries as I tried to clean the cottage. My mother watched as I scrubbed a coating of black filth out of the refrigerator and shower, and cleared piles of little plastic bags of rotten trash off the kitchen counter. An old mattress, ancient clothing, bundles of newspapers, and boxes of paperwork crowded the living room. Between this garbage, Mom had left a narrow path, like a trench.

In her downstairs bedroom, the extra twin bed sat covered with a pile two feet high of empty cookie packages and rinsed-out ice cream cartons, each item bagged individually in a clear, plastic gallon-sized bag and sealed with a twist tie. Now, I suspect that for some time she's been eating little more than junk food. I don't have the knowledge yet to know that this hoarding, and her food choices themselves, may be serious symptoms.

Outside the cottage, leaves and pine needles partly hid mounds of empty bottles and cans that Mom dropped over the steps rather than carry to the recycling bins in the boathouse. When the landscape contractor I hired cleared away the multi-flora rose, burdock, and sumac trees that thrived on the neglected lawn, his workers rescued several pots and fry pans that Mom set outside rather than clean.

Mom said, "I can pack the trash in my backpack and walk it up the hill to the car and take it to the dump."

I pointed out that she had not done that in a long time, and the fact that she was suggesting it reflected how disconnected she was from what she imagined she could do and the reality. In my impatience I clipped my words. I felt I had to be blunt.

Now, on the phone, I remind her of the reasons to move to our home. "It'll be like a new beginning."

She's quiet on the other end. After a moment she says, "As you're talking, I'm remembering the reasons."

"And Dr. Gavin shares my concerns, too."

"I tell you, honey, I couldn't believe how old I looked in the mirror this morning—so much older than just a few weeks ago."

I take a deep breath and try to keep my voice upbeat. "We can start with a two-week visit, Mom, to see how it goes. I'm not kidnapping you forever." This is a lie. Ben and I have no intention of bringing her back to the cottage, no matter what happens. The lie slips out before I know what I've said. Mom and I always try to be honest with each other, but now I want to ease her fear.

"I bought you new towels and washcloths today. And Ben set up a computer for you. We'll get you a library card." My husband, a gentle and generous man, has agreed to have Mom live with us because he knows it's what I want. In the back of my mind, I also think it might be good for our children. Until I returned to work last summer, I was a stay-at-home mom, and at ages seven and nine, our kids are used to my undivided attention. Perhaps with Grammy at our house, Andrew and Morgan will learn that sometimes other people need more attention than they do. The focus of the family will shift away from them, and they will learn self-reliance. This notion floats into my head as if a long-ago lesson of my own.

"Oh, that sounds good," Mom says. "I don't know why I was so worried."

In the course of our three-minute conversation, Mom swings from anxious resistance to complete acceptance. She even takes some initiative.

"Why don't we go over my list of things to bring?"

There is one more very serious factor that may explain her behavior and my delay in acknowledging its seriousness: grief. We have both been shell-shocked by a recent tragedy.

Last summer, her only son, my brother, died without warning, and since then, Mom has looked frail, as if ready to relinquish her own tenure on life.

David was fifty-two, schizophrenic, diabetic, and alcoholic. He weighed four hundred pounds, wore his gray hair past his shoulders, and had a long, thin, gray beard. In the late 1960s, when he was sixteen and I was four, Dave left home to live on the streets of New York City and, as my mother would tell me years later, "to try every drug he could get his hands on."

For years, he lived in another city several hours away in a single-room apartment. He was never able to hold a job. When Dave was a young adult, Mom tried hard to get him into treatment and work programs. After years of effort, she decided that there was only so much she could do for him if he continued to drink. She realized from her own 12-step program that she could not help him if he didn't want to help himself.

Once a year, beginning when I was a teenager, Mom would drive me to see Dave and take him out for lunch and to a department store. Sometimes, we met Dave in the entrance of the county's mental hospital. He was skinny then with greasy brown hair. In the passenger seat of Mom's orange VW bug, he told jokes in his soft, gentle voice and jiggled his cigarette on his knee. I barely remembered Dave, and thought of him as a distant, troubled uncle.

Dave's ex-wife, Joanne, lived in her own room across the hall from him, and they looked out for each other. One morning, he didn't take his diabetes medicine and later that afternoon, after he lay down for a nap, Joanne found him dead. As he never forgot to take his medicine, Joanne thinks he neglected to take his medicine "on purpose." I can only guess how distraught he may have felt living the same life day after day for years and years, going nowhere.

Joanne had Dave cremated, and spread his ashes over the summit of his favorite city park. Mom and I visited Joanne but did not attend the ceremony at her church. I assumed that my mother would plan some sort of ceremony, too, for us. I did not yet realize that she was incapable of organizing anything.

Mom had already made her own funeral arrangements, some fifteen years earlier. She told me she wanted to be cremated, and that she envisioned that I would hold a simple celebration of her life at the cottage. After Dave died, I thought more about how important it is to appreciate and take care of family. Why "celebrate" a life after it's over? Why not help make that life as good as it can be while the person is still alive?

Moving In

In early March, we move my mother into our home. The snow has melted, so we could drive down her road and bring a few pieces of her furniture to the spare bedroom off our kitchen.

A few days later, I help her pack. To my surprise, Mom seems happy and calm; I half expected her to change her mind at the last minute. As Mom searches for the dog's leash and muzzle, a box of tissue, and her sunglasses, I hold my breath, anticipating her frustration with packing, or her annoyance with me standing there, waiting. But she seems fine. Trinka, Mom's ten-year-old miniature Schnauzer, growls in her tiny, gray kennel cab amid the piles of recyclables in the living room. She's muzzled to prevent her nonstop barking. The dog is unused to other people and I've always been a bit afraid of her.

Then—another horrible discovery. Thirsty, I look for a gallon jug of drinking water in the refrigerator or cupboard and find none. Mom usually filled old milk cartons with free spring water from a spigot outside the local supermarket.

"I don't do that any more," she says. "I just drink the tap water."

My stomach flips. Pumped from the end of a pipe about thirty feet off the shale beach, the lake "gray water" is filtered but intended only for secondary use such as cleaning, not for drinking. I imagine an invisible broth of algae, fish scales, and gasoline.

"When did you start drinking the lake water?"

"I don't know. I've been doing it for years."

I wince. I might have noticed this a long time ago, if I had been paying attention.

Later, Mom pauses in her rummaging and smiles at me from across the kitchen. "Thank you so much for doing this for me."

"It's okay," is all I can think of to say. A fog thickens in my head, much like the cool mist on the lake outside her window. This fog is a familiar feeling, a kind of dampening, a fuzziness that softens my brain whenever I'm plunging into a major change in my life. I recognize the feeling but don't stop to think about what I'm doing. I want to help my mother but I have no real plan. My eyes flicker across the table at her and I manage to return her smile.

Almost immediately, when we stop at the dog groomer's house where we are going to leave Trinka for a few days, it hits me that I don't really like being in charge of Mom's life. A "what have I got myself into?" feeling washes over me. This is it. I'm taking Mom away from her own life, her own territory, her own friends. I'll be following her around, helping her, waiting on her—forever. Introducing myself to the groomer, I try to hide behind my mother to show this old friend of hers that I do not consider myself in charge of my mother—not yet.

The groomer, who has known Mom for twenty-five years, whispers to me when Mom turns away, "I've been worried about your mom for a while now. What you're doing is a good thing." With sad, kind eyes, she smiles and pats me on the back.

"You're a good daughter."

I find myself wondering why this groomer, or any of my mother's other friends, has never looked up my phone number to call me and express their concern.

When we arrive at our house, my seven-year-old daughter, Morgan, greets us. She's wearing her purple party dress and ivory tights with silver butterfly barrettes. She and her dad have baked a chocolate cake and decorated it with vanilla frosting and written in green icing, "Welcome Home Grammy." Andrew is off playing with friends. Mom gives Morgan and Ben a big hug.

Mom seems to like her lilac-painted bedroom. She has a private bathroom with a shower, her favorite framed photos, her radio for NPR. I've made up her bed with a new purple and mauve quilt.

The first thing Mom wants to do is unpack, ever so slowly and carefully, and designate specific places for her comb, brush, socks, checkbook, dog leash, tissues. I hover in her doorway. "Can I help?"

"No, sweetie, it's fine. I'm just getting organized." I want her to look at me, to include me and talk with me, but she looks down at her work. I want her to stop being so particular about *things*.

It's not a good omen that, within an hour of her arrival, I already wish she were different.

She lines up her bottles of medicine along the top of the bureau. She insists that she can still keep track of her own medication and I do not question her.

Mom stops for a moment to admire the view out her window into our tiny front garden. "When I sit at my desk," she says, "I'll be able to watch the neighbors come and go!" I smile because that is exactly the image I've had of her—sitting at her desk, working on her bills, gazing at the garden and neighbor houses as she used to watch the lake from her desk at the cottage—not as breathtaking a view, but something. I picture her at her desk or reading in bed, just as she did for much of the day at the cottage.

When Mom looks out her window she can see a cluster of four or five of our neighbors' small houses and the common space between the houses with its picnic table, cherry trees, rhubarb garden, and large, round boulders for kids to climb. Our community lies in the middle of old pastureland eight miles from the city. Parking is set away from the houses to leave the common areas pedestrian-friendly and safe for children, and we enjoy a large pond where we swim and ice skate. Though sometimes mistaken for a commune, our community is middle-class; many residents hold advanced degrees, and we represent a wide range of personal and spiritual philosophies. We are teachers, professors, computer programmers, musicians, stay-at-home parents, consultants, social workers, carpenters.

Ben and I first learned of this community in a newspaper article back in New York City. We were outgrowing our tiny co-op on the Upper West Side and longed for a college town where we could raise our children. A city boy, my husband felt nervous about moving to the "country." Ben was born in Hong Kong and raised, since age six, in Manhattan's Chinatown, then Brooklyn and Queens. He was willing, though, to do anything to keep me happy. Ever since our daughter Morgan's birth, I'd been struggling with post-partum depression. I wasn't sad or unable to function, but I felt sudden waves of rage. By the time we considered moving, I felt much better on an anti-depressant.

I was drawn to the intentional community's acres of open space, which reminded me of my childhood in the Adirondack Mountains. I'd never lived in suburbs and wanted to avoid them, and this community combined the best of the country with the best of the city. I was intrigued, as well, with the possibility of truly knowing my neighbors. Ben liked the fact that the college town attracted an international crowd and he wouldn't be the only Asian. He was less interested than I was in the social aspects of community, but he supported me in making the move.

Now I realize that, when I first moved here, I thought of the neighborhood as one large entity—a kind of parent, a mother figure. I assumed I would develop close relationships with almost all of the residents, that we'd each help and support each other. For the first few years, I worried constantly about fitting in with the other parents, making sure our children got along with the other kids, and contributing our share of time to the needs of the community.

Now I hope that Mom will make friends here and go out to lunch with them on occasion, but I don't expect my neighbors to take regular shifts to keep her company. I suspect that whatever Mom needs, I will have to provide myself, or arrange for her, using as many resources in town as I can find. Will I be able to manage it? I think so, but at this point, I am still innocent of the realities. I will soon realize that her care will demand far more.

Problems at Home

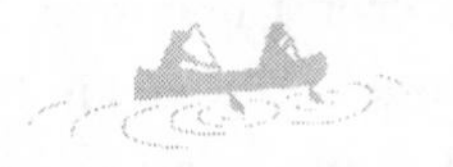

After four days, Mom and I are already getting on each other's nerves. Mom barely eats. Ben and I make a delicious stew for dinner, but when I stand outside her door and ask her to come out, she says, "Go away."

Trinka is an immediate problem: Mom lets her in through the back door onto the carpet without wiping the dog's wet paws. More serious: When the dog nips at my little girl and her friend, Mom says nothing. She sits in a daze.

"Mom, you need to discipline the dog."

Mom grabs a newspaper, rolls it up and starts whacking the dog.

"Mom, stop. When I said 'discipline', I didn't mean beat the dog."

She lowers the paper.

"Maybe we can lock Trinka in her crate when there are kids visiting," I say.

Mom shakes her head and scowls. "Trinka lost all her manners at that kennel."

"No, she acts this way because she's been living alone with you at the cottage for ten years. She's not used to being around other people, around children."

Mom is silent. Later, she goes into her room and refuses to come out for dinner. I knock, then open the door.

"Is there a problem, Mom?"

She's lying on her bed reading and doesn't look up.

"You."

There's a silver lining. When we snap at each other, I retreat to the hutch in the dining room where I store piles of laser paper printed on one side, and a stack of half-empty spiral notebooks. In the ten years since graduate school, I've written nothing, but since Mom moved in, I find myself scribbling on these scraps of paper. I hide notebooks in every room and carry one in my backpack to write on the bus on my way to work. They are my emotional safety valve.

As our lives continue to interweave, my first rule is Danger Control.

My first task: Take away Mom's car keys.

I'm worried that, while I'm not looking or I'm at work, Mom will walk out to her little green Honda and try to go shopping for cigarettes or chocolate, or maybe return to the cottage. I have to tell her that she should no longer drive, that I can take her wherever she wants to go. I dread this conversation. I fear her anger and indignation.

I knock on her bedroom door and find her reading, lying on her bed. She's mad at me again. Rather than come in, I stand in the doorway to tell her the bad news.

Mom looks up from her book and her eyes shoot darts. "Who says I can't drive? What makes you an authority on whether or not I should be driving?"

"I'm not an authority," I admit. "Dr. Gavin was very concerned about your driving."

She glares at me, unconvinced. I try another tactic. "As your only child, your only family member left, it's my unpleasant job to tell you that you can no longer drive." My words are formal and stiff. I want her to have sympathy for me as the person bearing bad news. I've read online that if you make it clear to a person with early-stage dementia that their behavior affects you, that it makes things more difficult for you and causes you stress, they are more likely to cooperate. I'm trying to be good at this.

Mom sighs.

"Plus, the traffic in town is awful," I hasten to add.

For the past ten years she's hated driving in city traffic. I don't tell Mom the real reason she shouldn't drive: her inability to be aware of the drivers around her and to make quick decisions. People in the early stages of dementia negotiate the road only out of habit. I don't need to spout facts, as it turns out.

"You're right," she says. "I don't want to drive in town." She shakes her head and looks down at her book. "I'll never find my way around." With another sigh she picks up her keys from the bedside table and holds them out to me. I step in and take them.

"Thank you," I say, and wait a moment. There's more to say, and I dread her response to the next step: "Will you let us cancel your insurance and take off the plates? Will you let us sell the car for you?" I doubt she's ready to let go of the car itself, the symbol of her independence.

Mom rolls over to face the wall. "That's fine."

Her easy acquiescence both relieves and frightens me.

• • •

The following weeks unfold like a test, one that both Mom and I are failing. Mom seems depressed or angry, no longer perky as she was on her first day here. I wonder if she looked forward to moving in with us because she thought I would give her my undivided attention. Maybe she feels neglected, ignored, judged, put down? I don't know, and for quite a while, I don't ask. I'm so accustomed to thinking primarily of myself and my husband and children that I can barely feel this seismic shift in my mother's world. It never occurs to me that her mood is perfectly normal for someone who has lost almost everything from her old life. I never ask a key question: *How would I feel in her place?*

Five days a week, I work from 7:40 in the morning until 1:40 in the afternoon at a nearby university as an administrative assistant and editor. I return home at 2:30 after meeting Morgan and Andrew at their school bus stop. In the mornings, Ben gets the kids ready for school and drives them to the school bus at the end of our road.

I worry about Mom sitting alone all day, and in the beginning I focus on making sure she gets enough to eat. For Mom's breakfast, if she gets up before Ben leaves for work, he asks her what she would like; if she's still asleep, which is usually the case, he leaves her some of whatever the kids had for breakfast and hopes that she will reheat it in the microwave. Before I leave for work, I find leftovers that Mom might like to eat for lunch, transfer them to a plate, cover them with plastic wrap and, before placing them in the front of the refrigerator, write "Mom" on a sticky note.

By the end of our first month together I suspect that she's not eating enough; she tells me she didn't like the food, or that she got so caught up in her paperwork she "forgot to eat." At first I blame this forgetting on her obsession with her bills, on her single-mindedness. I don't see this as a glitch in her short-term memory. I blame her personality.

I try ordering Meals on Wheels. Mom tastes one delivery—meatloaf with potato puffs and over-cooked spinach—and declares it awful. I ask her to try a few more of their meals—"Maybe we started on a bad day," I say—but the next morning she manages to find their phone number and calls to cancel.

In our tiny house built for energy efficiency, the kitchen, dining room, and living room flow together as one L-shaped room with little extra seating for another family member. Ben's favorite place is a desk tucked into a tiny alcove under the stairs at the far end of the living room—his "lair" we call it—where he plays video games and surfs the Internet. My favorite place to sit and snack or do paperwork is the dining room, a few feet from the kitchen, in the one chair that directly faces the pond through our large picture windows.

As soon as Mom moved in, she began to spend hours rooted in my chair, with her bills, a glass of ice water on a napkin, tissues, pens, a hairbrush, and the dog's leash covering half the table. To my surprise, she converted this space into her new desk instead of using her bedroom desk with the view of the garden. When I'm home, I ask her to please not sit in my favorite chair, and she's patient with me. She tries to remember to sit in the chair to the left, which still has a partial view of the pond, but she forgets. Wearing her nightgown, she reads and rereads her mail and munches on cashews or a stash of chocolate bars she keeps in the freezer. Though she's willing to clear off her belongings for our family meals, after work and on weekends I miss this space for myself.

• • •

When she's not at the dining room table, Mom wears her nightgown or only a T-shirt and underwear, and reads in bed, lying on top of the covers, half sitting, half lying down, her shoulders and upper body propped up on one elbow and leaning toward the lamp on the bedside table. She tells us she wants to help us out around the house, and tries a few times to set the table and wash the dishes, but to find everything she needs to do the job—or to remember how to do it—seems to exhaust her.

Her only other action is to head out the back door with Trinka and sit on a flat rock on the low wall of the raised bed under the maple sapling, where she smokes and grinds a bare circle in the grass with the butt. With the hand that holds the leash, she scrunches the collar of her navy-blue jacket close to her neck. For an hour at a time, she'll stare off toward the pond or the hills in the distance. Beneath her gray knit hat, her hair and face shine white in the cool spring sun. When I watch her through the window I'm startled by the whiteness of her hair, the paleness of her face, the curve of loneliness in the hunch of her back.

I start to search for activities for Mom, not quite knowing where to begin. Our neighbor Rita, the only other member of our community with Alzheimer's, goes to an adult day care program for people with dementia three days a week on the local van service for the elderly. I print out the schedule and show Mom the program's activities. She takes one look and refuses to go, declaring it "kindergarten." She's right; coffee and discussion, walking for exercise, crafts, and listening to books read out loud do seem much too simple for her. Rita's dementia is more advanced, and I've watched with pangs of pity and fear the decline of this vital, avid gardener into someone who needs constant supervision. Her children have hired aides, and other residents visit her regularly. There is a lesson in this—but I don't learn it until later.

I do send out an email seeking neighbors I can pay to visit Mom a few hours a week. Lydia, a psychologist who is currently a stay-at-home mom, offers to come by for three hours on Tuesdays and Thursdays. In the meantime, some of our retired neighbors graciously offer to take Mom into town with them for dinner and concerts. At first, she's excited to join them, but then calls these kind neighbors at the last minute to cancel.

It turns out my mother will not be making new friends and arranging to go out with them on her own. When I realize that she won't, or can't do this, it hits me for the first time just how poorly she's functioning. While the frightful state of the cottage didn't convince me of the seriousness of her decline, this does.

As an introvert, I long for time alone to recharge and relax. All day, my job requires me to listen carefully to my boss, coworkers and clients. When I get home I'm accustomed to time by myself when the kids go out to play.

Now I usually find Mom sitting at the table waiting for me with paperwork to go over, bills for me to explain. Sometimes she has written notes to remind herself to ask me something. I coach her through each step to write and record the checks and address the envelopes. One day, I help her fill out the paperwork for a new Medigap health insurance policy so she can see local doctors. I soon learn that if we spend more than an hour going over paperwork, or even just talking, we are both exhausted and snarky. As I listen to her talk on and on, as I explain the same thing again and again, my shoulders scrunch up, my breathing grows shallow; I want to jump out of my skin, the wooden chair feels so hard. After a few weeks of this, I learn to say at the end of the hour, even if we're not done, "Mom, that's all I can do for today."

Later, as I clean or cook, Mom asks me questions every few minutes. "What is this? Is this new? Has Trinka been out for a walk? Has she been fed? Do you have any ice cubes, my dear?"

As soon as I can, I retreat behind a book.

When I come home from work one day, my mother hands me another note that she wrote to remind herself to ask me a certain question. "Have you and Ben taken over my money?" she asks. "I haven't gotten a bank statement in weeks. The only thing I can think of is that the two of you have cleared out my bank account."

A wave of heat scalds my cheeks. "We just had your mail forwarded, Mom," I say. "You've only been living with us for three weeks!" I do not yet understand that dementia makes the confused person come up with strange, off-base explanations for what they don't understand or can't remember. My head is spinning, full of static, my chest feels heavy. How can my mother accuse me of stealing her money?

I arrange for a volunteer from the "Check It" program at the senior center to meet with Mom at our house while I'm at work, to go over Mom's bills and checkbook. When I try to help Mom balance her checkbook, she blames her confusion on my calculator. The woman from Check-It manages—I'd love to know how—to convince Mom that she can no longer keep track of her checkbook on her own. But when I ask Mom if the volunteer will come back, she smiles at me and says, "You can just do it."

"Are you sure?"

"Yes, honey. I've tried and I just can't make sense of it any more." She leans back, gestures to the newest pile of paperwork on the table, and then slumps down onto the arms of the chair. "I'd appreciate your help."

As soon as a stranger—not me—showed her how she could no longer balance her checkbook, Mom could let go of this essential piece of her autonomy, and accept its loss.

After that, we institute a new procedure: I open her bills, write and record her checks, and just have her sign them. I feel both relieved that I don't have to explain each step to her, and nervous because I'm taking on more responsibility for making sure that her bills are paid.

More problems surface: Ben, Morgan, and I all have asthma, and cannot tolerate cigarette smoke. Though we repeatedly ask Mom to please smoke outside, she sneaks cigarettes in her room. For fifty years, she's smoked up to two packs a day. She's tried many times in the past to quit, but without success. When she lived at the cottage, I convinced myself somehow that she wouldn't fall asleep with a lit cigarette and set the place on fire. Years ago, on an overnight visit, before the garbage and recyclables piled up, I remember standing in her bedroom door while we said good-night, and watching her deliberately snuff out her cigarette in an ashtray before she switched off her lamp. Here in our house, I'm uncertain she's as careful. One night at midnight, her puffing sets off the smoke alarm. She seems chagrined and stops for a few days, but then starts smoking again. I can't tell if she's forgetting our request or being stubborn. The smell infuriates me, and I have horrific visions of the house going up in flames.

When my neighbor Lydia starts to come over for a few hours two days a week, my mother just wants to talk to her, saying she has no interest in food. I feel relieved to have Lydia there to reheat the meals and gently insist that Mom try some of the food. But I'm also happy that they go to the library together and out to lunch.

They sit in the backyard on the rock wall and talk while Mom smokes. They go for short walks.

Mom adores Lydia, calls her "an angel who fell from heaven."

Lydia tells me, "I love being with your mom. She's such a sweetheart!"

Though part of me wants Mom to feel pleased that people appear out of nowhere to enjoy her company, another part of me wants credit and appreciation for making it happen. I know it's petty, but I tell Mom that I was the one who asked Lydia to come and visit. I remind her that we're paying Lydia by the hour out of her checkbook. The thought of another woman my age, a kind of substitute daughter, enjoying all of Mom's smiles and laughter twists a sour knot in my stomach.

A neighbor of mine, whose mother in another state has Alzheimer's disease, tells me how helpful she's found our local Office for the Aging and its caregiver support group. If she hadn't told me, I would never have guessed that there existed such groups as an Office for the Aging or caregiver support. In fact, I don't yet think of myself as a caregiver, but only as a daughter. I'll learn later that part of the reason why so many caregivers do not seek support is because they don't see themselves as caregivers; they don't recognize the label, or the fact that caregiving is a job, a new role in their lives for which they need information, support, and services.

At work I'm fortunate to have flexible hours, which allow me, on the following Tuesday, to leave work early to attend my first support group meeting downtown. Seven of us meet around a large table in a cramped room in the basement of a county office building. The facilitator, Dan, is a soft-spoken man in his forties whose mother had early-onset Alzheimer's disease in her fifties. Most of the tired-looking people around the table are at least sixty, wives or husbands taking care of their spouses at home. Only two of us are adult children caring for our parents with dementia, and we are both women. I am the youngest in the group by about fifteen years.

The people around the table take care of loved ones with Alzheimer's disease, vascular dementia, Parkinson's disease, and other causes of memory loss. When it is their turn to introduce themselves, some have to cry first. Many of the loved ones with dementia are in nursing homes or assisted living facilities; a minority lives alone in their own homes.

We talk about elder care attorneys; I learn that I should find one soon in order to become Mom's power of attorney and health care proxy, and help her complete a living will. We talk about how driving and the checkbook are the hardest things for people living with dementia to give up; I feel lucky that my mother did not put up a fight about driving and that she surrendered the checkbook.

We talk about whether or not to ask our loved ones' doctors for one of a handful of prescription medications that are supposed to relieve some of the symptoms of dementia temporarily (for up to three years). (See Appendix B.)

The next time I see Mom's doctor I ask her if Mom should take one of these medications, and she tells me that she's not sure they work, and at this point, the damage has been done. I agree with her about the damage having been done, but I regret having missed the opportunity five or ten years ago to convince my mother to give a medication a try. It never occurs to me that Mom might still benefit from trying one or more of these medications, and I don't know enough to research this further.

Dan also recommends the book *The 36-Hour Day* by Nancy Mace and Peter Rabins, a classic guidebook for dementia caregivers.

Someone else gives me the name of a good local psychologist specializing in elder care issues. We talk about how the county's

Family and Children's Services offers free caregivers' counseling in people's homes, and I make a note to call them.

The other women in the group ask me questions I cannot answer: "How are you doing? What losses are you feeling? What are you giving up to have your mom live with you?"

I have no idea what I've given up. I simply haven't thought about it. Yet. I know that I've been feeling overwhelmed, but at this moment I feel vaguely smug; unlike the other daughters in the room, I take care of my mother under my own roof.

One woman says pointedly in my direction that if her mother-in-law, who has dementia, were "held captive" at their home instead of staying at her assisted living place, she would go crazy. "She needs social contact and daily walks outside, and is happy there," the woman says. I'm not holding my mother captive, I think to myself; I'm just trying to make sure she has everything she needs. Inside I sneer a bit at the idea of assisted living; I assume that this woman is just rationalizing her family's decision to put her mother in what I assume is a cold, impersonal facility.

The women remind me that caregivers need to take care of themselves. Yoga is good, they say, so is tai chi. One woman says she developed heart problems when she was caring for her husband at home. Another gets the flu when stressed by caregiving. A daughter tells me, "We all think we are superwomen and can do everything, but we can't." A seventy-year-old woman, who placed her husband in a nursing home because she was no longer able to care for him in their home, tells us, "Human beings are finite. You can only do so much."

I listen, but their words don't sink in right away. My life motto has always been, "Pile it on me." Nothing has felt too difficult if I pushed myself hard enough. I don't realize my limitations are fast approaching. Soon, I will have to make a choice.

Instinct

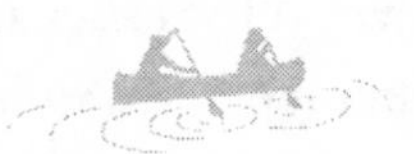

More problems surface every day. My mother has one contact lens, an old-fashioned hard lens that she's supposed to wear in her right eye. She's never worn glasses, only contacts. The hard lens is easy to clean—it requires only a rinse in saline solution, no disinfection—but soon I find the dirtied, shriveled lens in its dried-out case. Mom is literally turning a blind eye, and, metaphorically, so am I.

Mom and I drive to the cottage to get more of her belongings. I've convinced her today to wear her contact lens, but when we approach Silver Lake she says, "Is this my lake? It doesn't look like my lake."

Startled, I grip the steering wheel tighter, and fear this is the rapid deterioration I have just learned can happen: Is her long-term memory vanishing along with her short-term? Is this proof that she does have Alzheimer's disease and not just mild dementia from tiny strokes? Will her dementia progress like Alzheimer's disease? Will she soon be unable to dress, use the toilet by herself, walk, and feed herself? Will she end up curled in bed unable to swallow or move, eventually unable to breathe?

So far, her new primary care doctor has avoided the word "Alzheimer's." She told me, "It's the dementia that concerns us, not the diagnosis." At this time I don't know enough about how Alzheimer's disease is diagnosed, or the benefits of early diagnosis, to press the point. (See Appendices A and G to see what I learned years later.) The doctor did give Mom a brief neurological test, and Mom did not know the date, the month, or who was president, and could not draw the numbers and hands of a clock.

As we drive home from the cottage, and dinnertime approaches, I suggest a restaurant supper. She insists instead that we stop at her old supermarket for a half-pound bar of chocolate. In the car she proceeds to eat almost the entire bar.

"Won't that spoil your appetite?" I say.

Mom says, "That sounds like a judgment!"

This exchange escalates until I'm raising my voice and she's calling me a controlling bitch. When we get home, I head straight upstairs to my bedroom to cry. A half hour later Mom climbs up the stairs, sits on the edge of my bed, and offers a hug. I'm surprised that she remembers our argument; I thought her short-term memory loss would erase it.

"I'm sorry for acting that way," she says.

"I'm sorry, too. I'm sorry if I sounded condescending." I realize that my talking to her as if I'm her mother is not the best thing for either of us. I can't just take her under my wing as if she's one of my children. It won't be that simple.

"It's all right," she says. "I love you so much, and I want you to know how much I appreciate everything you're doing for me. You and Ben."

"I know, Mom. Thanks. I appreciate that."

When my mother apologizes like this for her half of our arguments, when she reaches to embrace me as I am, that's when I feel closest to her, when I love her the most. For much of our lives, she'd blame our arguments on me. Only when I was in my thirties did Mom begin to try to understand my feelings and her contribution to our rifts. Maybe it was her new anxiety medication, maybe it was the progression of dementia, but slowly she mellowed. If she hung up on me, she'd call back and apologize, or cry in relief when I called back. If I told her I was angry, she would listen to my reasons without argument.

When she offers this comfort, my mother is coherent and clear-eyed and beautiful. She's the mother who, despite our battles, has always shared her wisdom, encouraged me and loved me in her own way. I no longer feel mad at her. In this moment, I want to help her, give her things, create experiences she will enjoy.

I learn that I cannot spend more than two or three hours at a time doing errands with Mom—not because she's always unpleasant, she's not—but because everything we do is in such slow motion. She denies that she has much memory loss or confusion and wants to take the lead. Sometimes she welcomes my help; sometimes she bats me away. Concentrating like this for several hours leaves the synapses in my own brain singed like strands of hair in a flame.

It doesn't help that when we go out around strangers, Mom is charming and friendly. It's only when we are alone that she's negative and low-level sarcastic. The world receives her best behavior; I get her fatigue and frustration.

In late April, eight weeks after she moved in, Mom calls me at work at 9:30 in the morning to tell me that she's in pain. She says she got up earlier in the morning to use the bathroom and saw that her forehead was bleeding. Since she didn't want to wake me, she went back to bed. When she got up later in the morning, after Ben and I had left for work and Andrew and Morgan were in school, her head and the side of her chest hurt.

I rush home to take her to the hospital. She can't remember how she hurt herself. I assume she rolled out of bed in the middle of the night and bumped her head on the nightstand on her way down to the bare wooden floor.

In the E.R. Mom needs an X-ray of her ribs and a CT scan of her head. She enjoys all the attention and wants to laugh at herself, but laughing gives her sharp pain in her ribs.

"Don't laugh, Mom, lie still." I smile at her from my chair at the side of the hospital bed where I sit clasping my hands in my lap. I see myself as her sidekick; I'm only with her to keep her company while she talks directly to the staff herself. The doctors will decide what to do and Mom will either agree or disagree with them. I have no opinion and feel no urgency to ask a lot of questions.

A young female doctor swings in to tell us Mom might have a tiny rib fracture; there is nothing to be done, it will heal on its own. After Mom's blood work, I wander the hallways to find melted ham and cheese sandwiches for lunch. We eat, laughing that all the doctors and nurses seem to be blond ("Why is that?"), and her side feels better. We are both giddy with relief.

In the evening, Ben and I rush-order a bed rail online, a white, metal bar narrow enough to allow her to easily get in and out of bed, but far enough up the side of the bed to keep her upper body from rolling out. Each day before the bed rail arrives, I worry that I'll find Mom unconscious on the floor.

Going to the office is a vacation compared to being at home. When our neighbors comment on our having to take care of Mom's dog, too, I reply with a laugh that taking in a dog is nothing compared to taking in your mother.

As I rush about, I tell Ben, "The first ten years were all about the children; the next ten years will be all about Mom. I'll catch up with you when we're fifty!"

At noon on a Saturday, Mom's still sleeping in and I start to worry. She had coffee at five o'clock in the afternoon yesterday and, according to Ben, who stays up late every night, she couldn't get to sleep. I'm frustrated because I don't know what Mom can decide and control and what she can't. Doesn't she know that if she has coffee late in the afternoon it will keep her up all night? Can't she remember this from one day to the next?

When she lived at the cottage, she'd tell me over the phone that her pattern was to go out and do errands one day, be unable to go to sleep that night, then sleep in most of the next day. Often I'd call her around noon or in the early afternoon only to wake her, and she'd have no idea what time it was. I don't want her to get back into that night-owl habit at our house because it would be impossible to schedule any activities for her, and it would upset everyone's rhythms. If Mom sleeps most of the day, she will miss our meals and we'll have to fix meals just for her; if we hire more caregivers for her during the day they may be unhappy to find her still in bed. Lydia is perky and full of energy, and because Mom likes her, Lydia's able to get her up without a problem. Other caregivers might not have that luck; they might discover that when Mom has slept either too much or too little, she can be snappish.

I can see that it is hard, exhausting work for Mom to live with her memory loss. I should be more patient. What is my role here? To house her with all her quirks and let her keep her own hours, no matter how difficult it becomes to live with her?

After only two months with Mom, I start to imagine what her life might be like at an assisted living facility. She'd be expected to keep to a schedule, with a time to get up, take a shower, have breakfast, and take her medication. I bet they'd be even less flexible than I am.

Meanwhile, our home care situation worsens. Every day, Mom retreats to her room at the slightest perception of insult. Sometimes she appreciates my help remembering things, but other times she gets angry and tells me to mind my own business. She tells me she feels like "a piece of shit in the corner."

One day, in hindsight, I'll realize that during these months Mom lives with us, she is firmly in Stage Four of Alzheimer's disease—moderate cognitive decline. She can no longer handle many complex tasks, and she's increasingly moody and withdrawn.

Mom and I sit in the office of a psychologist who specializes in elder care issues, the woman recommended to me by my caregiver support group. At first, Mom resists; she doesn't see why she might need the advice of a new doctor. When I tell her that I could use the advice, she agrees to go. She sits in silence, with her ankles crossed, one hand resting on the other in her lap, a good girl in school. Forgetting our fights, she tells the psychologist that she's happy living with me.

"It's not always that happy," I tell the psychologist. "I know this is an unusual situation, but I want help to make it work."

The psychologist, a tall and slim woman with the cool air of preternatural calm, says, "Most adult children do not take care of their parents in their own homes. But I admire your effort. I want to help."

I tell her that I'm afraid I'm acting "dysfunctional" because I'm putting up with old dynamics between my mother and myself by having her live with me.

"I don't like the word 'dysfunctional,'" she replies. "I've seen it over and over again that adult children have an almost instinctual need to take care of their elderly, frail parents." She smiles. "When we see that our parents really need our help to survive, something almost parental kicks in. I do believe it is built in, biological, instinctual."

I feel so grateful to the psychologist for saying this I could jump up and hug her. I needed to know that my impulse to protect my mother was normal, understandable, maybe even beyond my conscious control. I'm relieved to hear that sometimes other adult children act on the same instinct and turn their lives upside down. We certainly lug baggage, my mother and I, but by living together, we've tried something most adult children don't even attempt. I feel proud, and I feel hopeful.

And yet, back at home, as my mother sits at the dining room table and crinkles the newspaper open and closed, sipping her glass of ice water, I just want to get as far away from her as possible.

Our History

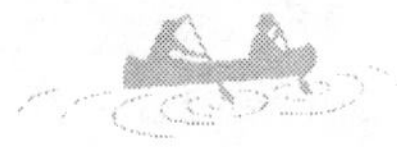

My relationship with my mother has always been complicated. While there may be no "normal" families, ours was more idiosyncratic than most. This fact contributed to the late diagnosis, and the delays in my own comprehension of my mother's condition.

Mom told me years ago that her doctor had encouraged her to give up teaching at age forty-nine because her depression and anxiety were getting worse. Two years before that she'd put herself into treatment for alcoholism, and she needed a chance to work on her sobriety. She'd been a heavy drinker most evenings since before I was born, possibly to self-medicate.

As a teen, I'd cook dinner and wash the dishes while Mom sat in our living room drinking White Russians. Sometimes, she'd pass out on her bed before dinner was ready. She was not a mean drunk; she just sat there every night in her cream-colored upholstered chair, with her ankles crossed on the matching footstool, lesson books and papers to be corrected piled on her lap, a dark anger in her eyes matching the cloud of cigarette smoke around her head. Sometimes I'd sit on the couch opposite her chair and do my homework—I was a top student, a self-motivated nerd. Instead of talking to her, if I felt annoyed about something I'd glare at her with my "evil eye," as she called it.

My mother was authoritarian—her word was law; I knew that she'd tolerate no anger or back talk. I'm not sure what the implied threat was, but it worked. A handful of times when I was younger, if I defied her or misbehaved, she would spank me with a wooden spoon. In the heat of the moment she'd smack me once on the bare bottom, leaving a stinging red oval. Once, when I was a teenager, she slapped me on the face. She had told me to sweep the basement stairs, one of my weekend chores, and I refused to do it immediately. We argued, and she hit me. I don't remember her apologizing, but she did look shocked at her own behavior. My memory of these few incidents left me afraid to challenge her.

Mom told me years later that she was never comfortable with teenagers; she preferred younger children—that's why she never taught above the fourth grade. Teenagers, she told me, could "see through" her, and that made her nervous. When a teacher asked me who my role model was, I said I did not have one, but my mother was my "anti-role model." I promised myself that I would never grow up to be my mother.

Even after she stopped drinking my mother intimidated me. She later called those years her "dry drunk" period. I see now that part of the reason I left home as soon as I could was not only to get away from her, but to prove that I didn't need her, that I could be independent.

In her first decade at the cottage, my mother flourished as a member of the small nearby community. She once again practiced the clarinet she'd played in high school, and joined the town band; she played a Hungarian princess in a theater production; she served as secretary for the local library's women's study club. In addition to volunteering as a master gardener, she studied landscape architecture and painted watercolors of pine trees and sunsets. She cross-country skied and did water aerobics. She worked part-time, first as a receptionist at an alcoholism counseling center, then as an alcohol education coordinator, and as a clerk in a bookstore. She continued going to 12-step programs, and invited her sponsors and friends to the cottage for visits. One of her closest friends, a Mennonite who lived on a neighboring farm, would drive her horse and buggy to the top of Mom's road and walk down with her five children to swim fully clothed.

Photos from that time show my mother carrying an extra thirty pounds. When she stopped drinking, she at first lost weight, but she soon replaced alcohol with a craving for sugar. The weight crept back on, most of it around her belly (a risk factor, I'll learn much later, for Alzheimer's disease) and her thighs.

Over the last ten years at the cottage, even though her diet remained high in sugar, Mom lost all of the extra padding of middle-age and became slim again. I will learn later that weight loss can be one of the first warning signs of Alzheimer's disease. Studies show that such a drop in weight often happens years before other symptoms appear, and results from the earliest effects of Alzheimer's on the brain.

By age fifty-nine, Mom had to stop working, and started to receive Social Security disability payments. Her depression and anxiety worsened to the point that she could no longer maintain even the most basic of jobs. At her last job, at the bookstore, she was so anxious and nervous she kept making mistakes at the cash register. She started to retreat from her community activities and stayed home. She also started to act obsessive-compulsive, though

I didn't know enough at the time to recognize her classic behavior. I simply knew that she could be fussy and uptight. Before she left the house she would spend a half hour picking each speck of lint off her clothes; she'd wash her hands frequently throughout the day; she'd spend days at her desk typing her monthly budgets on her IBM Selectric and then, with a ruler, underline expenses in red, income in green, and long-term expenditures to be saved up for, like roof repair or a new car, in black. Typos and slips of the pen merited a narrow strip of correction fluid, a half-hour's wait to let it dry, then crisp reconstruction of the missing digits. One summer when I was in my twenties, she hired me to paint the cottage, and she kept track of my wages in columns on graph paper, again in multiple colored pens, down to .0916666 cents per minute.

In the last years she lived at the cottage she covered her desk with sticky-notes to remind herself of tasks and appointments—"Phone Martha," "Feed Trinka," "Doctor, Tuesday 4:00." Although this habit may have been obsessive-compulsive, I know now that many people with early-stage dementia leave notes everywhere to help themselves remember things.

According to her medical records from Dr. Gavin, a psychiatrist had her try Nardil and Depakote for the depression and anxiety, but the drugs never seemed to help, or they gave her noxious side effects such as shaky hands. For the last few years, Effexor seemed to have smoothed her anxiety and lifted her depression.

During the time period when she tried these medications I lived hours away from her, and on the phone and in letters Mom would sketch only the briefest description of her struggles—to spare me, I think, from worry.

I wonder now if Mom was living then with the very early stages of Alzheimer's disease—Stage 1, "normal functioning," and Stage 2, "very mild cognitive decline," as described by the Alzheimer's Association, or Stage 1, "preclinical Alzheimer's disease," as described by the international workgroup led by the Alzheimer's Association and the National Institute on Aging. No one noticed, but the disease might have been starting.

In 1997, when Mom was sixty-five, both Dr. Gavin and her psychiatrist noticed some confusion and memory lapses. A CT scan of her brain showed mild damage, probably from tiny strokes. A neuropsychological exam at a medical school two hours away reported "minor word finding difficulties, somewhat slowed information processing, and diminished sustained attention." According to their report, Mom had spoken to her doctor and psychiatrist about her concern that she'd withdrawn from all social activity, stopped cleaning the cottage, spent too much time on her paperwork, and felt overwhelmed by any decisions involving money. The report also mentions that Mom had a few incidents with her car that I didn't know about, such as minor fender benders, and being stopped by the police for weaving. Her sleep was erratic, and she had trouble concentrating on tasks such as following recipes. She showed "mild depressive symptoms characterized by sadness, irritability, fatigue, ruminative thoughts, and decreased decision making."

Because of her "excessive attention to detail and orderliness," the evaluators found her to have obsessive-compulsive personality disorder. And in her "rapid, excessive speech" they saw evidence of "hypomania." On the phone Mom would talk on and on about how I should invest in mutual funds, or, when I visited, what groceries we should buy for our meals, and often I could not help but insult her by looking away or huffing in impatience.

When the evaluators had called to ask me how I thought my mother was functioning, I told them I had noticed that she had difficulty remembering how to buckle her seat belt. And I was "concerned about her judgment," according to the report, after an incident the year before when my mother took the bus to New York City to visit Ben and me and one-year-old Andrew. She had offered to baby-sit while Ben and I went out for dinner, but then left Andrew alone, toddling around the apartment, to go outside and smoke. That day I was more than concerned, I was livid.

Their exam concluded that her primary problem was not a "neurodegenerative dementia such as Alzheimer's disease," but her obsessive-compulsivity and hypomania. At that time, they thought my mother could still live alone.

Looking back, I can see that, despite the exam's conclusions, Mom had passed Stage 2 of the Alzheimer's Association description of the disease—very mild cognitive decline—and was most likely in the beginning of Stage 3—mild cognitive decline. Though the symptoms were minor, she showed the tell-tale difficulties of finding words, performing tasks, planning, and organizing.

In the last five years my mother lived at the cottage, Ben and I and the kids stopped visiting the house itself because we knew the cottage was so cluttered there would be no room to sit down or eat a meal together. Mom would meet us half way at a restaurant, or she'd drive to our house. She also never let any friends indoors. Her best friends, Bill and Susan, owned a cottage two doors down from her, yet when they came over she'd chat with them outside on the chipped concrete steps.

On one rare evening when I visited the cottage, I found her sitting at her desk working on piles of paperwork. The bulb in her lamp had blown, and she hadn't been able to figure out how to replace it. Perched on a ream of paper and folders on the corner of her desk was a slender, flickering candlestick.

Frayed

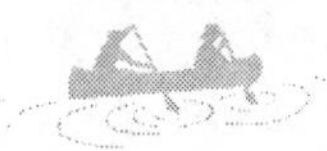

It's late April in 2005, and my mother may sound and act like an adult but is now, in essence, my third child. I would like her to function as an autonomous adult, but she can't. She doesn't want to be dependent on me, but she is.

We argue again one morning before I leave for work. When I returned to work after a being a stay-at-home mom, I hired a housecleaning crew to come in every two weeks. Today I ask Mom to get out of bed before the cleaners arrive at 9:00. I want them to be able to get into her room and her bathroom. She refuses to get up.

"I'm paying for the whole house to be cleaned," I say. "If they can't get into two of the rooms there isn't much point in having them come."

Mom glares at me. "You're so bossy. So manipulative."

"And you're stubborn, Mom." My voice rises and I say a few more things I regret before leaving to seethe in the car. I feel angry and depressed all day.

At the kitchen table, later in the evening, we talk. Mom felt bad all day, too.

"I feel guilty for being such a pain...when you've done so much for me," she says. "I know I can be difficult." She starts to cry. "I don't want to go back to the cottage."

I get up to hug her. "It's okay. I want you to be happy here."

"I've felt so scared. I've felt worse...the past couple of months."

"I know, Mom."

"I think I should stop smoking. I know I shouldn't smoke in my room." She adds, "I think the cigarettes are affecting my memory."

Yes, I think to myself, they might be, but it's too late now. I'm impressed, though, with her willingness to quit.

"How about we don't buy any more after this?" I say.

"Okay, honey, let's not."

I'm feeling more positive, but my little girl, Morgan, no longer likes Grammy living in her house. She tells me that Grammy tells her what to do, to clean up after herself, and not always in a nice way. The tension between my mother and my daughter seems to echo the stress between my mother and me when I was a child. As Mom's anxious perfectionism and her drinking used to push us apart, Mom's dementia will prevent her from learning from her mistakes with her granddaughter and from growing closer to her. She will forget what upsets Morgan and be unable to avoid the same patterns in the future.

Andrew, on the other hand, does not seem to mind Grammy, maybe because he had more of a relationship with her when he was a toddler, before her memory got worse; the two have a connection that Morgan and Grammy do not. Andrew remembers sleeping over at the cottage with Grammy by himself when he was three years old. Mom set up her pup tent on the front lawn next to the steps and squeezed the two of them inside. Andrew remembers that night fondly, even though, around four in the morning, Mom told me later, she climbed out of the tent and went inside to her own bed, leaving Andrew alone in the dark. Andrew woke up with the rising sun and managed to find Mom inside, apparently without feeling scared, but I was incredulous.

I call Family and Children's Services to see if one of their counselors can come talk with Mom and me about how things are going. FCS has a small division to support family caregivers with counseling and respite. They can send a volunteer to stay with Mom for a few hours while I get away, but as I already get out of the house every weekday to work, I don't need respite. I need more people to talk to who understand the stresses of caregiving.

Mom and I meet with an FCS counselor in my living room. She suggests the Adult Day Program and the city's Meals on Wheels, and I tell her Mom rejected both. The counselor says I am already doing many good things for myself (the support group, the psychiatrist, hiring Lydia), and congratulates me. Mom has little to say. I take the counselor aside and tell her that I'd like to meet with her a few more times, alone. "That's fine," she says. "Our main concern is you, the caregiver."

In early May I attend a presentation at work called "Elder Care." I'm fortunate to work for a large university that hosts a wide range of life-balance workshops for its employees. Dan, the facilitator of my Alzheimer's caregivers support group, leads the presentation. He explains what basic ADL's, "activities of daily living," are: eating, bathing, dressing and undressing, toileting, continence, walking, and transferring (getting in and out of bed or a chair, for example). I note that at this point my mother needs no assistance with ADL's. Except for her short-term memory loss, and the beginning of long-term memory loss, she is in pretty good shape.

Dan points out that many people mistakenly believe that either Medicare or Medicaid will pay for their long-term care needs when they age. Medicare, however, pays only for short-term medical care—hospital stays under 100 days, rehab, and limited at-home care and therapy to recover from a short-term illness or injury. When you stop getting better or stop making improvement in rehab, Medicare ceases to pay. Medicaid, on the other hand, a joint federal and state program with much variation from state to state in requirements and benefits, will pay for long-term care, but only when you've drained your savings and become impoverished. Until you've "spent down" your assets, the only way to pay for assistance with long-term care such as bathing, dressing, and toileting is out of your own pocket or through a private long-term care insurance program.

My mother doesn't have long-term care insurance, and never talked to me about it. I doubt she would have felt that she could afford the premiums. In any case, it's not clear to me if she would qualify for benefits. Most long-term care insurance will start to pay benefits when the person needs help with two to three ADL's, and Mom needs help only with "instrumental activities of daily living" (IADL's) such as shopping, cleaning, and transportation. However, most policies will also begin paying for care if the person's doctor determines that they are "cognitively impaired" and in need of frequent supervision to ensure their health and safety (for example, assistance with cooking so they don't go hungry or leave the stove on). In that case, Mom would likely have qualified for a part-time aide even when she lived at the cottage.

But I won't understand any of this clearly for several years. I will look back and remember those plastic-wrapped plates of food that sat untouched in my refrigerator, and I'll realize that Mom ignored them not because she was distracted but because she could not remember how to work the microwave, or even how to find the food or follow the instructions on the sticky notes. I will realize that my mother was already cognitively impaired when she lived with us, and I will come to forgive myself for my denial. Even as dementia shares my table, my home, I fail to see.

The tension between us increases and our exchanges soon take on the form of bickering. Mom and I argue over small things—how much dog food Trinka should eat so she doesn't get fat, why I read a book instead of listening to her complaints—and the bickering escalates into the increasingly common ending of my mother locking herself in her room.

One night, I knock on her door and call "Dinner time!"

Through the door I can hear her say, simply, "No."

"Is there anything on your mind?" I ask.

"I don't want to get into it right now."

Living with my mother means that I must watch what I say, my tone of voice, my expression, to avoid condescension. I feel as if I'm a child again, reading her face as she drank. *Is she in a good mood, or is she angry with me? Have I done something wrong?* Now, I resist falling back into that habit. I stay away from her as much as possible. I remind myself that I am human, that I cannot always react with grace.

Finally, I snap. We are driving home engaged in another endless petty argument. "You need to mind your own business," Mom snaps. "You can never keep your mouth shut."

My breath grows tight. "You know, Mom, you don't appreciate the work I do for you." I exhale sharply. "Maybe, if you think I should mind my own business...maybe you'd be happier living somewhere else." This is the first time I ever suggest that she move. In this moment I know in my gut that I cannot do this any longer.

I grip the steering wheel tighter. "I can't be a martyr, Mom, and live like this. It's not fun, you know, not knowing when you'll think I'm being helpful and when I'm going to piss you off."

As my voice climbs higher Mom falls silent, shrinks down into the passenger seat, and stares straight ahead.

What I don't realize yet is that Mom and I clash partly because I'm still using reason to explain things to her. I speak to her as if her short-term memory is intact and she can follow a logical argument. It will take me awhile to master more artful ways of communicating.

When Mom moved in with us I never imagined that I would become not only the main provider of her food, shelter, clothing, prescriptions, medical appointment schedule, and transportation, but also her primary source of entertainment and social engagement. I finally begin to realize that coordinating my mother's life is a part-time job in itself, and one for which I am not qualified. I could hire a geriatric care manager to oversee some responsibilities for Mom, but they cost anywhere from fifty to two hundred dollars an hour, and I'd have to supervise what they did anyway.

Mom may be better off, feel less like a "piece of shit in the corner," if she lived somewhere else, with me visiting often but not being in the middle of her life every day.

At my caregivers' support group, Dan says that when people with dementia move to assisted living it may allow them to conserve their independence longer. "Moving into assisted living might free them up," he says. "It may lift them out of burdens they no longer want." In my home Mom seems to carry the burden of feeling unnecessary and in the way. But if we tried assisted living, would I be trading one kind of guilt for another—guilt about being so tired of listening, about feeling profoundly bored hearing the same things over and over, for the guilt of leaving her alone?

If Mom continues to live with us, will Morgan suffer because Grammy gets annoyed with her? Will my relationship with Ben suffer because of the daily stress of Mom and me butting heads? He's been keeping out of our way as much as possible, but in his own home, how long can that last?

I meet with a social worker who helped me several years ago when I struggled briefly with the post-partum depression. I tell her I suspect that having Mom live with us was a bad idea. The counselor says that she's concerned not only about my stress level but also about my daughter; living with my mother could affect Morgan's self-esteem over the long run if Mom is grumpy with her, telling her what to do.

"It's all right to have your mom live with you for now," she says. "You had to do something. But not for the long-term."

I know she's right, but I feel a twist of panic over the uncertainly of what will happen next.

In a staff meeting at work I'm close to tears because I feel so overloaded at home I have to turn down our department's director when she asks me if I'd be willing to take on additional work. Normally I get bored easily and ask for more responsibility than my job requires, but now I tell her, "I'm too worried about my mother. I can't take on anything extra. When things settle down, you know I will step back up and do whatever you need." In the back of my mind I'm thinking of my boss's "family first" policy, how she told me when she interviewed me that, in her department, family always took priority over work. And beneath my boss, the assistant director is a woman who lost her mother to Alzheimer's disease. I feel both embarrassed that I'm falling apart, and determined to assert my need for less pressure. I'm lucky at work to have these two women who understand.

I attend another class on caregiving sponsored by the Office for the Aging. Dan, the facilitator from my support group, leads the discussion again, and I nod in recognition when he talks about the effect of caregiving on "life balance." He says, "adult children of aging parents recognize the shift in their role more quickly than do spouses or partners caring for each other. Adult children are more likely to question the effect of their caregiving on their life balance and to recognize stress." Yes, it has taken me only three months to "question the effect" of caregiving on my life. An arrangement that seemed logical to me at first now feels destructive for everyone.

Family Week

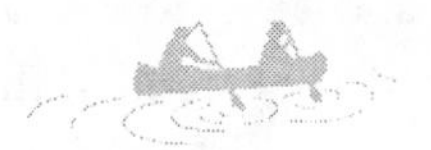

I've read that we tend to remember the bad things that happen in our lives while the good things dissolve into mist. As primitive humans remembered the colors and patterns of poisonous snakes, our modern brains tend to recall moments of pain and sadness more easily than pleasant memories because we are hardwired to try to avoid those situations in the future. I'm sure my mother and I spent time together in my childhood that was pleasant and loving, more than I remember. I know that when I was a baby she was an early member of La Leche League and nursed me until I was two. I know, because of my father's mental illness, that my mother was forced to support our family, that he was abusive to her, and that each afternoon after her teaching job she would find refuge in cuddling with me. I know that when I was four, and she married my stepfather, Mom took me swimming each summer at a "secret" swimming hole in the Adirondack woods, and held me on her lap in the sun. I know that when I was five and six she gently knotted my wet, freshly-washed hair at night in white socks to make it curly, brushed it in the mornings into pigtails, and tied ribbons in bows around the rubber bands. I know she read me nursery rhymes and fairy tales from the *Golden Treasury of Children's Literature*, and sang to me, and taught me to bake.

Those good memories do not stand in the foreground. I remember instead a dreary atmosphere, shades of gray like my stepfather's old farmhouse, filled with unhappiness. Bats once flew through my second-floor bedroom, mice and squirrels lived in all the walls, and moles burrowed up through the floor inside the cabinet under the kitchen sink. I was afraid to go into the kitchen at night lest I see the moles' tiny beady eyes looking up at me. In my bedroom, the ancient, stained floral wallpaper peeled off in sheets.

In the outside world, my mother flourished. She worked at the local elementary school as one of the first special education teachers in the state. She loved the freedom of being a pioneer in a new field, and the intellectual challenge of creating her own curricula from scratch.

When I was in third grade, my mother left my stepfather and rented a ski cabin in Vermont, where the two of us lived by ourselves for my third-grade year. She found a job teaching at the school. By my fourth-grade year, Mom and my stepfather must have reconciled because we were back at the Adirondack house.

The summer before my sixth-grade year, Mom and I packed our belongings and moved over two hundred miles to live with my grandfather, his new wife, Laura (my grandmother had died three years earlier), Laura's eighteen-year-old son, and her elderly mother. My mother and I shared a queen-sized bed in their tiny house and tried to stay out of the way. I did not know it at the time, but my grandfather was dying from lung cancer and heart disease.

A few months later, my grandfather died and left my mother enough money for her to buy the two of us our own house two doors down, with new furniture and wall-to-wall powder-blue carpeting. Mom took a job teaching special education in an elementary school the next town over. Later that same school year I had to move back in with Laura and her mother by myself, temporarily, when Mom went to the hospital for a radical mastectomy. At forty-four, she had found a lump in her right breast. She told me years later that she found satisfaction helping the other women in her breast cancer support group. She never spoke to me, though, about her mastectomy, and ten years passed before she would let me glimpse her scar.

Mom was forty-six when she had herself committed to an alcoholism rehabilitation program in St. Paul, Minnesota, one of the best in the country, she said. She would be gone four months. I would stay with Laura again. Mom asked me to sign an official form from the center saying that if she left the program early, or if she ever picked up another drink, she authorized me to have her sent back to the center. I had just turned fourteen.

Toward the end of her first month at the rehab center, the program directors asked me to fly to St. Paul on my own for "family week." I was the only representative of our family. I was not allowed to see Mom by myself; I had to go in with a counselor. In a small room with yellow curtains on the one window, a gray tiled floor, and black, metal chairs, Mom sat on one side of the room, I sat on the other, the counselor in the middle. Mom was to begin by listening, not talking.

"Martha, tell your mom why you feel angry at her," the counselor encouraged me with a smile. "It's okay."

Whew, I thought to myself, this man has no idea what a huge request that is. As I searched for something to say, her face relaxed but her eyes burned brighter, flaring like a lighter.

Finally I said, "You never listen to me. You're always angry about every little thing I do. You're always right and I'm always wrong." Hesitating, I added, "You don't let me talk back. One time I tried to talk back, when I didn't want to sweep the basement stairs, you slapped me." I don't remember what else I might have said; my heart was pumping too fast for my brain to store the words.

When it was my mother's turn to talk, I could not hear. My anger had unearthed itself and expanded to fill the room like a mass of thorny vines, leaving no space for me to listen. I already knew that she found my behavior annoying, that I angered her. That was nothing new, after all, but my speaking up for myself—my "talking back" and being listened to—was momentous. This meeting proved to be the first step of what would be years of struggle and growth between us.

After the in-patient treatment program, Mom was required to live in a halfway house in St. Paul for three months. She had to attend 12-step meetings every day, and walk two miles each way to a full-time job in a factory (what kind of factory it was, I don't know). I still have a six-page handwritten letter that she wrote after one of her shifts. A portion reads:

Dear Martha, my Honey,

I waited every day for your letter to come. I was so hurt and disappointed each day not to find it. Then today it was here!

My roommate's alarm went off at 4:45 this morning. I jumped out of bed thinking it was mine, and she never woke up to turn it off. I was pissed, but I didn't tell her. I will have to tell her if it happens again. That's a little scary, or a lot scary, but I have to say things to people about my being angry. I've stuffed angry feelings all my life and have been a "good girl," and it's gotten me in a mess. The anger I used to turn on you was mostly alcoholic anger, brought on by the drinking or the need for a drink, and the great amount of my angry rage was built up from little angers not expressed during the day to other people, and then I blasted it all out at once on you. I am ashamed of that. I know how I hurt you that way...

I have to walk to work. It's a 25-minute walk and it's so damn cold and icy and snowy and rough walking and it's still dark, and I'm all alone and I hate it all. The factory is noisy and boring, boring, boring, and dirty, and it's hard to have someone to talk to because of the noise. It's doing the same thing over and over and over from 7:00 to 3:30. My mind begins to run on memories and wanting to come home and knowing I can't because I'm not ready and I'm told you need time away from me.

I know, I'm feeling sorry for myself. I have been so afraid that you had stopped caring for me, but your letter tells me that you do care about me and miss me and love me, and I am so grateful for your letter telling me all those things. I'm willing to take these three months to get better, but the kind of help I get here is not the kind of help you get at a hospital.

You had a taste of the kind of help I'm getting when you were in Family Week group. "Tough love" is what it's called—and it hurts and is lonely and confusing...

They say I have to hurt before I can change my behaviors that lead to my drinking so I won't have to drink anymore, but I feel so unsure of what I'm doing. I'm supposed to share my feelings by telling someone right away every time—that's the way to get better and stay better. I find it hard to feel anything, know what I'm feeling, and say it.

I wish I had you here so we could both practice all this together so we could be really close. I hope you will get into your recovery program so you will be into sharing your feelings with me when I get home.

You are such a great girl. I am so proud of you in many ways...I love you so much and want to be close to you always. You are the most important person in the whole world to me.

Kisses and fuzzies,

Mom

I don't remember receiving this letter, but I'm sure that, at fourteen, I would have felt baffled by my mother's feelings. I certainly would have recoiled at her desire to "share" her feelings with me when she returned. Deep in adolescence, I was too far into myself to meet her halfway in recovery. Then, when I left home at sixteen to go to college, we lost any remaining time to practice new ways of being with each other.

I wish I had found this letter years earlier. I would have understood better why my mother felt it so important in my adulthood to express her anger right in the moment, usually without self-reflection to temper it. I tried to support her in her need to speak truthfully and to care for herself, but the constant expression of her displeasure felt as if she was dumping her feelings on me—and she didn't necessarily want to listen to my feelings in return. Only in my early thirties did I press my mother to hear my side. I encouraged her to think about why she felt angry before she expressed it. For a few years, she tried. Then the dementia started, and much of the patience and insight she gained was lost.

For fifteen years, she went to 12-step meetings for alcoholics and adult children of alcoholics, and then counseling.

As a teenager I followed my mother to my own 12-step meetings for family members of alcoholics. In those church basements, I learned that I was not alone, that other kids had the same experiences, and that I was a separate person from my mother with a right to my own feelings. I learned that, as a result of growing up with an alcoholic, I had built up my own defenses and backward ways of dealing with people. In these groups I also found support and encouragement in the stories of others. In the presence of people from all walks of life leaning over their coffee and hot chocolate, watching and listening intensely to each other, I first sensed a higher power.

As I grew into a young adult I pictured this higher power, God, or "Good Orderly Direction," as some in the program would say, not as an entity above us but as the grace I felt around those tables, soothing energy flowing like a radio wave from soul to soul, neighbor to neighbor, linking and uniting and amplifying the best parts of ourselves.

Tough Love

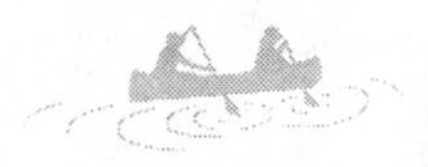

With my old journals, I find a letter my mother wrote to me after I dropped out of college and visited briefly:

I've thought about your idea that I don't like you, and what I think at this point is that what is happening is the natural pain (on both sides) of our separation in your growth toward independence. It's a normal, painful time for both of us, and perhaps it's taken us both a bit by surprise. It will take some growing time for both of us to establish ourselves on a new footing with you and I living our own separate lives with all the leaving of past ways of relating, and fumbling through the new. Remember here at the cottage after you interviewed at Elmira College last September, how it hit us that our past life together was ending? How we cried? What I didn't know then was that this separation would come in stages, and here we are at another one of those stages. I am crying now as I realize it. But, it must be—for both of us. It's so hard to let go of you. I guess it's a good thing we got as angry with each other as we did early this month—it forced the separation that has to come. I mourn losing you, though, and only hope upon hope that we can grow toward a new and good relationship.

It was awfully hard for me to have you just "stop in" last Saturday night and then leave again. You held yourself away from me physically and verbally as if trying to maintain that person who is you against an attack of my "mothering." But I was so glad to see you! I thought of how it must have felt the same way to my mother when I left home and then was a visitor. It's a wrenching that has to happen. And I do want to do it well, Martha, so that you'll keep coming back.

I worry about you off on your own, if I let myself think about it. It's hard to let you make your own mistakes. But it's the only way, I know.

Hope all is going well for you.

Love,

Mom

Should she have worried? Perhaps. At the time I was a part-time minimum-wage aide in an elementary school who couldn't afford a 30-cent box of spaghetti.

I wish that my mother had not given up so easily on our relationship. Sure, I was keeping my distance, but her hands-off attitude reminds me of the "tough love" she talked about in her 12-step program, the philosophy that to love me she needed to let me make my own mistakes. I know she meant well, but she took it to an extreme. As a young adult living on my own, I could have used a whole lot more guidance. Mom was never particularly nurturing, but I needed her to try. It's a wonder I survived those early adult years of not enough money, too many men, and too little birth control, without permanent damage. I fully intend to offer my own children more guidance when they become young adults, even if they resist.

At eighteen, I moved three hundred miles away to New Haven, Connecticut, with a boyfriend and fifty dollars. After three weeks, we broke up and I ended up sleeping on the couch of a man I met in a bar. I never called Mom to rescue me.

The one time I did call my mother to help me, it was right after I dropped out of college and had hitched a ride with a friend to work on a dairy farm in Pennsylvania. The dairy was run down, filthy, about to be closed by the health department, and when I realized that all the employees slept in one large bedroom with bare mattresses, I asked to use their phone. Mom drove down to get me but she seemed more annoyed than worried.

Over six years in New Haven, I held about two-dozen part-time and full-time jobs. I moved from rented tiny rooms swarming with cockroaches, to sharing nicer houses and apartments, to renting my own apartment on the third floor of a brownstone. On Thanksgiving, my mother would drive to see me and roast a turkey in the various cramped kitchens of my boarding rooms and apartments. More often I'd take the bus partway and she'd pick me up and take me to the cottage for a few days. We would argue, but the only anger allowed was hers. Once, when I slammed the car door behind me after an argument, she threatened to call the police. A few times she just kicked me out of the cottage. Without a car, I had nowhere to go and she'd drive me in silence to the bus station.

Mom would tell me that when I was angry the look in my eye and the tone of my voice "could be quite unpleasant for those on the receiving end." She was right, but I didn't give her much credit for saying it because I thought she had the same problem.

For Christmas the second year after I returned to college, when I was 26, Mom gave me a blank album with a note attached:

> *I hope you will use this album to hold copies of all the good things people have said about you.*
>
> *Then, on days when "Nobody loves me, everybody hates me; I'm going to eat a worm," you can open this up and remind yourself what a fine person you are.*
>
> *Love and kisses,*
> *Mom*

It's hard to stay mad at my mother when I can see that she loves me like that. I know she intends only good.

False Relief

By the end of May 2005, when my mother has lived with me for three months, I meet on my own with the psychologist. She tells me that the fact that Morgan hates having Grammy at our house "seals the deal": To protect Morgan's self-esteem, Mom "must live elsewhere."

She explains how difficult I might find it to arrange help for Mom, whether at the cottage, at the senior apartments in a nearby town, or here in the city. Arranging care long-distance, even from across town, would be really stressful for me, she warns: "Aides don't show up, the agency will be calling you all the time; you'll be on the phone left and right making sure your mother has all the help she needs."

I ask her where she'd recommend that Mom live and she says there are two assisted living places in town that can handle mild dementia. "Your mother can have a good life in assisted living," she says. "When you do get together you will be able to just enjoy each other's company."

I nod, picturing Mom and me going out to eat and to concerts, and how I could drop her off afterward into someone else's capable hands. Though I don't make a decision right away, the thought lightens my spirit.

Every development that follows makes the decision seem inevitable. Soon, my mother shows another stage of her deterioration—hostile reversals and more accusations.

Near the end of May she says, with a gleam in her eye, "I want to move back to the cottage. At least until next winter." Her voice is flat. "I'm tired of your constant negativity."

My stomach contracts; I can feel my pulse in my skull.

"Well, I've had it with your stubbornness and put-downs," I say.

With a deep breath, I race on: "If you move back to the cottage, your friends and neighbors there will have to make all the arrangements. They'll have to come here and move you back. They'll have to arrange rides for you. They'll have to find someone to shop for you and clean and cook. They'll have to make sure there's a railing on the footbridge.

"I'm not willing to help you long-distance, Mom. I can help you only if you live here in town."

As I spew all of this I know perfectly well that Mom cannot make these arrangements to move. She cannot plan anything beyond a phone call or two. There is no chance that she will go back to the cottage on her own.

Mom glares at me, then looks down at her book and waves me away.

At the computer I research "guardianship" on the Internet, in case Mom calls her friends and convinces them to help her return to the cottage. If she were to insist on moving, and I refused to help her, I would be keeping her here against her will. I might have to go to court to prove that she can no longer make these kinds of decisions for herself. I understand from my support group that my having Power of Attorney is insufficient; without guardianship I cannot stop her from trying to move back to the cottage.

I call Bill and Susan, Mom's neighbors at the cottage, to warn them that Mom might call them for help to move back there. I ask them to please tell her it's a bad idea. I tell them how she can't drive, shop, cook or clean for herself, how she can't pay her bills. "Of course," they say. "We didn't realize how bad it was."

After dinner, Ben and I talk for a long time. We decide that we've tried our best but it's not working. We will give Mom a choice and a deadline: She must make her own arrangements to live elsewhere, or try a "respite" stay, a temporary two-week visit, at one of the two assisted living places in town. We knock on her door then stand in her doorway together and tell her that she must decide what she wants to do within a week. We know that time means little to someone with dementia, but a deadline will tell Mom that she must make a decision soon, that she cannot delay. We tell her that we can help her visit the assisted living homes to see which one she likes better. Mom listens in silence, then says, "Just go."

Knowing that within a few minutes Mom will probably forget what we've said, I type a seven-page letter with all the reasons why she can't live at the cottage anymore, why it's not working for us to share a house, why she needs to try a short stay at an assisted living place. The next day, after reading and re-reading the letter, Mom says, "It makes sense." She's calm. I can tell she wants what's best for me and Ben and the kids. The letter helped her make her own decision and she's willing to visit the assisted living places.

I hope that, once she moves, she will forget that I said it was temporary.

• • •

I ask Lydia to go with Mom and me to tour one of the assisted living places. Another neighbor, Andy, who has always enjoyed Mom's company, comes along for our visit to the other place. Mom will feel more comfortable about her decision if someone else whom she trusts tells her they like the assisted living places.

One place, Greenway, is a non-profit in a well-maintained building overlooking the city. It includes both independent apartments and an assisted-living section with one-room studio apartments for people who cannot cook safely on their own and need help with meds and bathing. We find the staff friendly and inviting. Part of me, the part deep inside that still denies that my mother needs help, hopes that Mom will act normal enough during the interview to qualify for an independent apartment. But after talking with Mom for only a few minutes the director whispers to me, "Your mom will definitely need to be in assisted living." I feel let down, almost embarrassed, as if my mother is deficient.

Greenway brings in students from the nearby universities who volunteer with activities, classes, and cultural events. I'm a bit put off, though, by residents slumped sound asleep in chairs and wheelchairs along the main hallway in the assisted-living section, their heads sagging. Mom seems to be much more "with it" than these folks. I fear that if she moves here she will quickly decline.

The other place, Maple Grove, is closer to us, and is also homey and well kept with warm staff, many activities, and a view of a small lake. But it's private pay, without a sliding scale. If Mom were to move here and run out of savings, she would not have her rent reduced to fit her Social Security and teacher's pension as she would at the non-profit, but would be asked to leave.

When we arrive at Maple Grove, a young woman is playing the violin in the living room. I'm happy to see that the residents in the audience sit up straight with open eyes. Mom, Andy, and I look only at the main building at Maple Grove for people who need minimal assistance. Their smaller building next door is a locked "memory care" cottage for people with dementia. In my mind I picture the memory care cottage as a mini nursing home with brusque, overworked staff in white jackets, the residents alone in their rooms in the most advanced stages of dementia, bed-ridden or in wheelchairs, spoon-fed, unable to speak. I imagine stark white hallways, silent except for the occasional moan or piercing cry. When asked if we'd like a tour I just shake my head and mumble, "No thank you."

When we return to my house, Mom and I compare Greenway and Maple Grove. Their assisted living residences offer similar amenities: three meals a day in a main dining room, snacks, a library, a hairdresser, daily activities such as coffee and conversation, ceramics, concerts, and outings in a facility van. I prefer Maple Grove, even if it's private pay, but I don't tell my mother. I want this decision to be hers as much as my own, to respect what remains of her ability to choose her own life. As we talk, Mom forgets the details of each place, but remembers how she felt when she met the staff. She has always been sensitive to whether or not she feels an emotional connection with people. When she says that she likes the staff at Greenway better, that decides it for her, and for me. Greenway has only one room available, a tiny room overlooking the parking lot, but I know that it won't be empty for long. I fill out the financial summary, the social history, and the medical forms. I write two checks for Mom to sign: one for the first month, $2,400, and one for the same amount for the deposit.

At 7:00 a.m. the next day, before anyone else can ask for this room, I drive to Greenway and slip the completed application under the case manager's door. As I straighten, a wave of relief surges through my body. *This place is what Mom needs. What I need.* She can enjoy her own routine, her own space, and new friends, and I can hand over this daily responsibility of watching and helping her to a paid staff. I can return to a role I'm more comfortable with, behind the scenes—independent daughter visiting her mostly independent mother—a relationship I fully expect will be healthier for all of us and a great deal easier for me. Any guilt I feel about moving Mom into an "old age" home lies buried, at least for now, deep below this overwhelming feeling of relief.

Part II

ASSISTED LIVING

Small Indignities

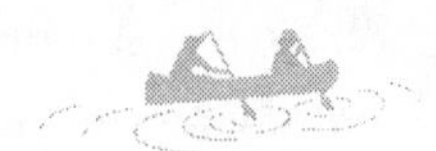

When Mom moves into Greenway, she has more savings than most Americans, thanks to a lifetime of pinching pennies. Upon her retirement from teaching on medical disability at age forty-nine, she realized that she needed to take charge of her financial future. She took a class on the stock market, and formed an investing club with a few women friends. For the next decade and a half, until she reached early-stage dementia, Mom studied the mutual fund reports called prospectuses (I remember that word because she talked about them all the time), and tracked her income, expenses, and investments each month.

According to Forbes.com, thirty-seven percent of Americans in 2005 have no retirement savings at all, and for those who do have savings, the median value is only $27,000. In June of 2005, Mom has $17,700 in her checking account, and a total of $121,500 in an IRA and mutual funds. Using her monthly income from Social Security of $882, and teacher's pension of $607, she will have to deplete her checking account by an additional $911 a month to pay for Greenway, plus $300 to $500 a month for Medicare and supplemental health insurance premiums, prescription costs not covered by insurance, dentist visits, haircuts, and clothing. I try not to think about how soon I'll have to dip into her IRA and mutual funds, or how many years her savings will last. Deep in my heart, I feel an acceleration—the meter is running.

I visit Mom about once a week; if I wait longer than that she chides me in a gentle tone: "I thought you'd given up on me."

"No, of course not," I say.

I don't hear in her words that she might feel lonely or even rejected. I just hear confusion. I remind her that I'm close by and will visit her often.

I drive her to all of her doctor's appointments, and her favorite thing to do afterwards is to go out for an early dinner or ice cream. Meals at Greenway disappoint her. Unlike the residents in the independent section of Greenway, as an assisted-living resident, Mom is not allowed to stand in line for the fresh vegetables and fruit in the salad bar; she must wait at her table for the same poor iceberg lettuce with tomato and cucumber or macaroni salad. I imagine this rule about the salad bar materialized because many assisted-living residents become confused and might take too long choosing which items they want, perhaps growing agitated, while the independent residents wait in line behind them. Nevertheless this rule is one of many small indignities. Another indignity is that staff members may open her door without knocking to tell her it's time to eat. When I notice a wooden chair in the middle of her room Mom tells me a staff member came into her room at six o'clock one morning while she was sleeping to change a light bulb in the dome in the ceiling, bringing the chair with her to stand on; not only did the staff person not ask permission to enter the room, she never finished the job and left the chair where my mother could bump into it.

At first, the staff assigns Mom to sit at a table in the large, main dining room with two other women and a man from assisted living. When I join Mom for a few meals, her tablemates pick at their plates with grave expressions in complete silence. Mom's social; she likes to ask people questions and to laugh. I can't bear seeing my mother trapped with such depressing company three times a day every day.

I ask Daphne, the case manager, if Mom can be moved to a different table. Advocating for my mother, even in this small way, feels risky to me. I don't want to develop a reputation right away as a bothersome family member. I fear the staff will resent my nitpicking and treat my mother less kindly, but soon I'm glad I spoke up. Within a week, Mom finds herself in a smaller wing of the dining room in the happy company of three talkative women from her assisted-living floor.

My mother seems to have forgotten that she ever smoked. Upon moving in she had to quit smoking cold turkey; their fire regulations require that residents walk twenty feet outside to smoke, and the staff does not have time to accompany the residents outside. This seems miraculous; she never seems to crave a cigarette, never even mentions her habit of fifty years.

For these first few months Mom has continued to take her medication alone in her room, one of only two residents in the assisted-living section to do so, Daphne tells me. Now, though, Daphne gently suggests, first to my mother and then to me, that it might be a better idea if Greenway kept track of her medication. Daphne and I agree that really we have no way of knowing for sure whether my mother remembers to take her medicine on schedule.

Apparently Daphne's patient manner convinces Mom to cooperate, and Mom relinquishes control of this with the same grace she did her driving, bill paying, and cigarettes. Twice a day, she will wait in line outside the medication room for her pills to be handed to her in a paper cup with another small cup of water to swallow. I feel sad picturing my proud mother waiting in line like a schoolgirl, but I'm grateful that Greenway can monitor her medication more closely than I have.

Before she moved in, the maintenance staff painted Mom's room ivory; the room looked fresh, with soft, clean carpet in a light rose. To keep my guilt at bay, I made her room more homelike, by hanging white, scalloped-edged café curtains to block the view of the parking lot and main entrance. The low, short curtains give her privacy but also allow an unobstructed view of the sky. I decorated with new brass lamps with ivory shades, and other items.

I left new wastebaskets in the bathroom and next to the desk, but found out later that the cleaning staff will not empty the trash unless someone—me, I guess—remembers to place the baskets outside Mom's door in the hallway. Right then, with the wastebaskets, I sensed that Mom might need more help than Greenway could provide. But I pushed this thought aside, assuming the trash rule was just a quirk in an otherwise reasonable system. Certainly Greenway must have other residents with mild dementia who might forget such a weekly task.

Mom and I enjoy each other's company more now that we're not living in the same house. Over lunch at a nearby restaurant, she is so excited that she just talks and ignores her food. As I listen to her, I notice for the first time in many years that even without makeup, my mother is still beautiful. This beauty was hidden by the gauntness of early dementia when she lived alone, then by her dark moods when she lived in my home. Today her smile is genuine—stunning—her laugh generous and usually directed at herself. Mom's eyes, once a blue-green speckled with brown, have turned the sky-blue of bachelor buttons, growing lighter and lighter each year. Her nose is slim, her cheekbones high. Her shoulders are narrow and bird-like; I imagine her upper body a lattice of little bones, featherweight.

Mom pulls from her lap a yellow folder bound in a thick rubber band, full of notes, she says, to remind herself of what she wants to tell me. I lean forward on my elbows, curious, but when she opens the folder I can see that the papers are ancient bills, torn-out pages of magazines, and junk mail. On top of the pile, she has clipped a few small pieces of notepaper. Her chicken fajita grows soggy while she reads her notes. Two college students, young women, she says, have talked to her recently. The first one interviewed her for an hour outside on a bench under a tree. They had an "easy rapport," Mom tells me, and though she doesn't remember what they talked about, she remembers how much she liked that young woman. The student will come back in four months to interview her again.

A second young woman interviewed her in a more formal manner, with less chatting back and forth, but encouraged her to write down four "commitments" for her health. Mom tells me with enthusiasm that she has promised herself she'll do the following:

1) Wear her one contact lens every day.

Great! I think. I worry that without the lens she will weave more when she walks, and fall. I realize now that Mom may have difficulty remembering the steps involved in putting in the lens. Today, though, she's wearing it—terrific! Such a small thing makes me feel so relieved.

2) Walk for exercise. The second student says she will return and walk with her.

I think to myself that walking is great. I'd love to see Mom use the wood-chip trail through the woods next to Greenway, but I worry that even walking around inside Mom might weave and fall. Will the student make sure she doesn't fall?

3) Make a dentist appointment.

4) Get a primary doctor.

The last two commitments embarrass me. Will this student think that my poor mother is abandoned at Greenway without a dentist or a doctor? Of course she has both.

"Your doctor is Dr. Claiborne, remember?"

"Oh, yes, I liked her. She mothered me. I'll take that!"

Dr. Claiborne came recommended to us by the elder care psychologist as someone who would give Mom her full attention. The psychologist's first choice was a geriatrician, but his practice was full. As in most cities, we have a shortage of doctors trained specifically to work with the elderly. Dr. Claiborne is not a geriatrician, but she listens patiently to Mom, looks her in the eye over her bifocals, touches her arm, and laughs with her.

Another day Mom tells me she has a new "best friend," another student from the college, a young woman from Egypt with whom she has shared bits of her life story as well as the name of her favorite shampoo. I feel a bit jealous of their conversations, as I did with Lydia. Mom tells me that the students who come over and lead activities, polish the residents' nails, or just sit and talk are "one of the two good things about living in that place." The other good thing is the friends she's made. She can't remember their names but she clearly enjoys their company. She calls one friend "the woman with the white hair." She's started to hang out with this friend and others at night to watch old movies on the big-screen TV in the main living room.

I feel unsettled when she tells me that she's reading less at night because "I have to watch these movies." How long will it be, I wonder, before she spends all of her days, as so many of the other residents do, in front of the TV?

After lunch, walking with me to the car, she turns to me with a smile and says, "Thank you for the repast, my dear. That's the right word, isn't it?" I agree that it is and we laugh. We both enjoy finding just the right word. I have been told that I speak as if I'm composing a short story in my head. I'm sure that comes from all the years of listening to my mother read to me as a child. When I speak or write I can hear my mother's voice, her cadence.

Often when we drive back to Greenway my mother says, "Oh, do I have to go back to *that place*?" Sometimes she calls it a hospital and the residents "patients." Sometimes she talks about the "children," and how poorly they're doing in class. I correct her and tell her that she's a resident, not a patient, that it's an assisted living place, not a school, but perhaps I shouldn't—she's right, in a way: It is more of an institution than a home.

A Fall

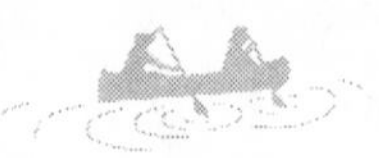

One week there's an art exhibit in the Greenway auditorium of photographs of women with breast cancer, some of them naked from the waist up. Mom strolls beside me, glancing at the photos with a mild expression as if she feels no personal connection. I stop myself from asking her if she remembers having cancer. If she doesn't remember, I don't want to know. That would be yet another sign that she's losing big chunks of her long-term memory, that her dementia is more serious than I want to admit.

A few days later, I take a day off from work as one of my two annually allotted personal days to drive Mom two hours to her preferred breast clinic for her annual mammogram. Mom's checkup is uneventful, but we have a bit of a mishap before the appointment. We arrive two hours before the appointment and decide to go out to an early lunch. Since our chosen restaurant won't open for another half hour, we walk next door in the strip mall to a clothing store, where we pass the time flipping through racks of blouses and pants. I don't yet realize that I need to walk next to Mom every second. We separate for a few moments, browsing in different aisles.

I lose sight of her, then hear her groan. I turn a corner in the middle of the store and see that she's fallen down a short flight of stairs. She lies crumpled on her side, her arms and legs flat and limp against the floor. One young clerk rushes over to help. Mom laughs it off and lets us pull her upright. She seems to be fine, no bruises, no cuts, no broken bones.

A few hours later, her left foot starts to hurt. When we get back to town she can no longer walk. I take her to the convenient care center where an X-ray shows she has a tiny fracture in her foot. As with her rib fracture when she fell out of bed in April, we are told that this fracture will also heal on its own. She will need to wear bandages and a boot brace for support, but won't need crutches or a wheelchair. The resident assistants (RAs) at Greenway will change her bandages, and Mom will be able to put weight on her foot and walk.

After Mom's fall down the stairs, I worry more about her weaving as she walks. When I take her out, I cajole her into holding onto me. I remind her that she fell and broke her foot.

"No, I didn't," she laughs.

"Yes, you did. Remember that brace you had to wear? It's on your desk.

"I'm not going to let you fall again on *my* watch," I say.

Mom smiles and wraps her arm around mine, or interlocks our fingers. Her hand is tiny and slim and warm. There is not much weight to it, but there is still a firmness of purpose, as if the only thing in the world she wants to do is to be with me.

• • •

Twice a year I treat myself to a weekend retreat for scrapbookers at a local hotel. I love having two whole days and nights to sit by myself. I immerse myself in trimming the photographs, remembering the stories behind them, writing the captions, and decorating the pages. The vellum sheets I slip over the finished pages protect the album from water, sunlight, and fire. I leave with something beautiful and permanent.

In October I finish a forty-page album about the cottage that I can't wait to show my mother on my way home from the hotel. The album is filled with photos of our family from the late nineteenth century through Mom's last years living alone at the cottage: earlier generations farming near the shore of the lake; later generations picnicking, bathing and rowing, fishing for trout, and steaming clams. One photo shows Mom at fourteen standing on the old dock, slim in a two-piece bathing suit, smiling coyly at the camera with her chin tucked into her shoulder. In others she's splashing off the shale beach with a plump baby David; holding me as a toddler on her lap on the concrete steps next to my grandfather; then sitting with me, a gawky thirteen-year-old. She's wearing her brown bathing suit and smiling at me as if amused, her legs tanned in the sun.

My mother's family has been going to the lake for several generations. Her father's parents, my great-grandparents, lived above the lake a few miles south and ran a small vegetable farm that supplied food for a private high school. They didn't own property on the lake, but they were allowed to visit the school's lake frontage. I have photos of my mother's parents when they were courting, picnicking with friends on the narrow beaches, shaded by the pine trees and maples on the cliffs. My grandfather, who grew up on the farm, bought the current site of the cottage in the 1950s.

Back then it was legal to extend your property out into the lake. Grandpa rolled rocks off the cliff behind the cottage to deepen the beach and build up the yard. He planted trees (the willow is still there, ancient and wide as a redwood), and built the railroad tie breakwall.

In 1964, as Grandpa used to tell the story, he woke up one morning to find "the sun rising in the wrong window." Cans of gasoline in the boathouse, a few feet from the cottage to the south, had caught on fire. By the time Grandpa ran up the hill to use the neighbor's phone to call the fire department, the cottage had burned down. A year later, when I was a year old, the new cottage was finished—not much larger than the old one, but solid and comfortable with its pine paneling, a fireplace, and picture windows. A set of drop-down stairs led to a new second floor and two small upstairs bedrooms, and I remember being scared for years of those steep, narrow stairs.

My favorite place to sleep was in the twin bed closest to the windows in the upstairs bedroom overlooking the lake. I'd crank open the windows and tuck myself under the musty wool Army blankets. The wild night air smelled of fish scales, seaweed, and miles of deep, roiling water. With yellow light from the kitchen glowing through the slit of the stairs, I drifted off to the lapping of the waves on the shale, the adults laughing below me, the clink of liquor glasses on Formica.

I arrive at Greenway with the cottage album to find Mom skimming a novel in the tiny, two-room library. She still reads, but has trouble remembering anything longer than a newspaper article. She often waits in the library for lunch and dinner to start across the hall. As usual, Mom greets me with a big smile, and her hair is brushed and neat, her bright pink sweater youthful-looking over her slim hips. She coaxes a friend to sit next to her and look at the photos with her. Catherine is a quiet eighty-year-old with flyaway brown hair and a lop-sided black headband, one of the women who share Mom's dining room table. The three of us sit at the only table in the library, me leaning across one side, Mom and Catherine together with the album between them on the other side. Mom points to each photo, and the long-term memories must come easily on this day because she explains the history to Catherine in the focused, teacherly manner she must have used with her students years ago.

Every few minutes, my mother cranes her neck to check the clock over the bookcase: She cannot be late for dinner at 4:30, she says, or "they will come looking for me." Dinner is so early for the assisted-living residents, I suppose, to make room later for the independent residents. Five more residents slip into the library, not to read but to sit, hands folded in their laps, in a row of chairs against the wall, to wait until the meal is ready. I glance over at them to see if perhaps they are enjoying my mother's little history of our family, but only one man is paying attention, and he looks annoyed. The others, all women, stare down the hall toward the dining room.

Will my mother end up like them? I wonder, waiting for dinner with nothing to do, no interest in reading, no reason to talk to anyone? At this moment my mother seems more alive than anyone else in the library—maybe, I imagine, in the whole building. She blazes like a cardinal in a flock of barn swallows.

Role Reversals

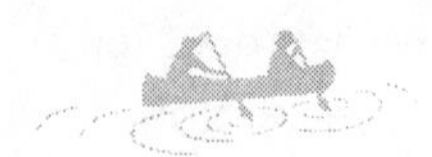

As the months pass and soften my memories of the stress and tedium of Mom's time in our home, the guilt I managed to bury when I moved her to Greenway begins to resurface. I start second-guessing myself. Is assisted living the best place for my mother to live? Have I abused my power to influence her decisions, consigned her to a hollow semblance of life? I never thought I would resort to segregating my mother from the rest of the community in an old age home. It feels like defeat, like giving up, and it nags at me.

In November, as an employee at the university I take an undergraduate writing class on "The Art of the Personal Essay." I quickly find refuge in writing, but also discover it can be a direct conflict with any extracurricular activities with my mother.

I call my mother to tell her that I cannot take her to visit the cottage today as I'd promised, saying, "I'm not feeling well and I have an essay due." I picture her sticky-note on her desktop calendar ("Martha, cottage"), and to make the call I have to fight an overwhelming surge of guilt.

Mom surprises me. She says, "That's fine, honey. Feel better."

Relieved, I return to my laptop. I tell my kids that if they interrupt me I will have to bite them. "Oh—in your thoughts," Andrew says. "That's okay."

When I am completely still except for my fingers tapping up and down on the keys, when I am completely absorbed by the process of writing, and hiss at Andrew and Morgan to be quiet, my only fear is that my children may remember me when they grow up as a frowning, snarling mother in an armchair, drunk on words.

Once, while I spend four hours writing an essay, Ben does all the work of getting Morgan ready for a sleep-over: setting up the tent in the backyard, inflating the air mattress, cooking dinner, making them a snack, walking Trinka before bed. At 9:00 he growls, "Why do *I* have to do all this crap?" My steadfast, mild-mannered husband does have his limits.

Another day, the dirty dishes are overflowing, the laundry is backed up, Trinka is leaking pee on the carpet, and Morgan is begging for a school friend to come over to play. I'm supposed to email another essay to my classmates by 4:00, but I don't feel like writing. The day before, I spent the meat of the day running errands with my mother. At my kitchen table, we went over her bills.

"I think it's time…for me…to hand the cottage over to you," she says.

"You already did, Mom. Last year. We went to the lawyer's office and you transferred the cottage to me."

"I don't remember." She looks as if she's about to cry.

Later she says, "I want to go home, but not back to *that place*."

With another prick of guilt I pretend I don't hear her. There's no point talking about "that place" again; Greenway seems like the only option. Another move might hurt her more than help her.

Ben can see that I'm exhausted so he offers to drive Mom back to Greenway. I hope that Mom won't mind my absence, but she says, "You're not coming? I need you. I want *you* to take me." She looks at me with a sheepish smile.

"You're like my mommy. I need my mommy."

My stomach twists. In that moment I don't want her to need me. I don't want to be the only one she wants. I don't want to do this anymore.

Her smile collapses and her brow wrinkles. "How awful…that you have to be my mother and I'm the child."

I take a breath, and feel my annoyance slip away as quickly as it appeared. I didn't think Mom was aware of this shift in our roles. I feel both gratified that she has finally recognized this shift, and awkward, embarrassed, as if I've been caught pretending to be something I'm not.

"No, Mom, you're still my mother, and I'm still the child." A quick dissembling, but, at the deepest level, true. I give her a weak smile and loop my arm through hers. I feel tender toward her again, and decide to bring her home myself.

As we walk up the path to the car she turns to me. "I don't know…how all of this…is going to work out," she says.

"I know, Mom." I'm at a loss for words. I stop to hug her and walk the rest of the way to the car with my arm around her shoulders. It's first time I've ever held my mother that way. Sometimes the only thing I will be able to do for her, I think to myself, is to be close to her, to touch her.

I drive her back to Greenway feeling fiercely protective and close to tears. In the dining room, where dinner is about to start, I find no staff members to give my mother a hug as they often do.

An RA appears at a distance and glances at us but doesn't say hello. Mom's tablemates fiddle with their napkins, oblivious.

Alone in a Crowd

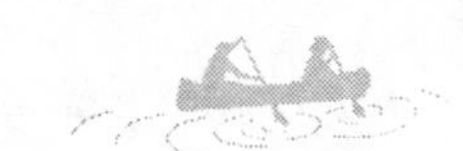

A year after Mom moves into Greenway, I extend the gaps between my visits from one week to two. Looking back, I'm surprised that I visited so infrequently. In these early years of my caregiving journey I am still in denial about the extent of my mother's decline, and still estranged from her. Each of us has been used to living separate lives, and once my mother settles into her own routine at Greenway, I return to mine. I make sure her bills are paid, drive her to appointments, and take her out for an occasional lunch, but the rest of the time I stay away. I convince myself that she has a full life with new friends, her books, the craft classes, concerts, movies, and visiting students. Though the "assistance" in this particular assisted living facility seems sparse, I assume that Mom is getting whatever daily help she needs. But is she? I don't know, and years later I'll regret this lapse in my vigilance.

Even though I resist visiting, when I'm away from my mother I fear that when I return she will no longer be there, that I will lose those parts of her—her sense of humor, her ability to find grace in any situation, her gentle laugh, her encouragement to "keep 'er cool"—that have mothered me even when I haven't felt particularly mothered.

On the other hand, it has been a peaceful year with Mom, a time to catch my breath.

The value of Mom's mutual funds has risen over the past year by $9,000. In April, I have to tap into the funds to continue to pay for her room at Greenway. I cash out $10,000, leaving her with $92,00 in mutual funds and $29,000 in her IRA. The meter is quickening and I dread the day we come to the end of her funds. What then?

In the fall I take my mother to a reunion of my father's side of the family. Mom's ex-sister-in-law, Nadine, will be there. Mom hasn't seen her in forty years but they used to be close friends. Nadine told me last year at the reunion that she can't wait to see my mother.

My father will not be there—his behavior with his mental illness is so disruptive that his second wife, now his ex-wife, has stopped inviting him. My half brother and two half sisters will be there with their spouses and children. Over the past twenty years, I've visited my half siblings only a few times, and my mother has never met them. We'll gather in a pavilion at a state park two hours away, the same place they held their reunions when my mother was married to my father. Part of me hopes that she will remember this place, the gorge and the waterfalls, and feel happy.

When I call the Greenway RAs to ask them to get Mom up early for the reunion, I expect it to be a short, simple call. Instead, Sharon, the head daytime RA, tells me she will "try" to get Mom up but "sometimes it's very difficult." And she adds that, oh, by the way, "We're having an awful time getting your mom to take showers. We don't think she's doing it on her own, and she won't let us help her with it." I agree that Mom doesn't want someone with her when she's naked. Last year, Mom called me in fear that one of the new RAs would "make" her strip and take a shower.

Sharon says that they are keeping track of whether Mom seems clean. "Maybe she's doing a French bath," she says, "like some older folks are used to doing." Your mom looks clean, she says. Have I noticed anything? A few times over the past year, I say, I've noticed that Mom smelled a little, but not lately. Sharon tells me as well that Mom refuses to let the RAs into her room to get her dirty laundry; they have to sneak in when she's out of the room, "because we have to get it done," and then Mom is grateful when they return the laundry. Yes, I know, I tell her, she doesn't like anyone coming into her room, and she forgets that she doesn't have to do her laundry herself.

When Sharon mentions the shower issue, I immediately feel a twinge of anxiety. I do not yet know that this is a typical part of the dementia progression. My mind starts working on how I can help the situation, what might happen next. I want to know about problems, but I don't expect to be told about my mother's declining ability to take care of her personal hygiene when I'm calling about a routine issue such as a wake-up call. I'd prefer that someone call me and arrange a time when I can talk.

"I wish I'd known about this before," I say.

"I'm sorry. I thought Daphne had already called you. Daphne really has a way with your mom, you know. Maybe she thought she could talk to your mom and get her to shower more often."

"Sure. That makes sense."

Daphne probably remembers how overwhelmed I felt when I first moved Mom into Greenway. I had asked Daphne to please handle as much as she could without asking me for help.

An example was explaining the rental agreement to my mother. Daphne spent hours going over the contract with my mother, again and again, because Mom always wants to understand paperwork even if it makes no sense in her brain. Daphne told me afterward that she had never before spent so much time explaining the rental agreement to anyone. I had told her that my patience for such matters was also exhausted.

Now on the phone, Sharon tells me about her own mother who had dementia, and was "much, much worse" than my mother. "I was always on the phone," she says. "Your mom is really doing very well."

I know she wants to reassure me, but I feel as if she's being condescending, as if I have little to feel stressed about and am being a bit of a baby. I measure the level of my anxiety about being my mother's caregiver by comparing my new role to our hands-off relationship in the past, not to how I might feel if her condition were to become worse in the future. I don't yet understand—how far and how fast will my mother decline?

My mother enjoys the two-hour drive to the park, but once we're there, hardly anyone talks to her, not even Nadine. Nadine is the same age as Mom but looks twenty years younger. One of my cousins asks me if Mom has Alzheimer's disease. I spend the afternoon holding my mother's hand to weave between the picnic tables, to make sure she doesn't trip on a table leg or a small child. I find her a warm spot next to the fireplace and bring her hot chocolate and plates of food. When Mom gets up to walk around and I grow tired of following her, I can see her talking with Nadine. Nadine smiles, points out the door toward another building a hundred feet past the parking lot, then turns away from Mom. I figure out that Mom is looking for the bathroom. As she heads outside by herself

I sprint the length of the pavilion to gently grab her arm and steer her around the broken chunks of sidewalk.

I leave disappointed in our relatives for ignoring Mom, but perhaps it's more of a challenge than I realize for people to connect with my mother. If I met a relative I hadn't seen in forty years or had perhaps never met, and they looked as pale and lost as my mother did today, I probably wouldn't go out of my way to talk to them either. I'd be nervous about what to say, perhaps even a little afraid.

The reunion makes me wonder whether something similar happens at Greenway when the independent residents mix with the assisted-living residents. I wonder if the staff encourages the two groups to interact or if they remain apart like boys and girls at a seventh-grade dance? Though Greenway has a new activities director, she serves the whole facility and can't possibly have the time to give the assisted-living residents the attention they need. For extra help, the facility relies on the student volunteers; in rare instances families hire private aides. Residents such as Mom, who shy away from activities, just sit in their rooms or watch TV most of the time.

One day, Daphne, the case manager, calls me to convey some of her concerns related to their annual report for the state. Her main concern is that when she does sign Mom up for activities and remind her of them, at the last minute Mom refuses to go.

"Your mom's dementia is no worse than several others' here," she says, "so I'm not sure what's going on."

She tells me that she's paired my mom up with a student again, but it has been difficult for the girl to see Mom because Mom sleeps late in the morning and reads in bed for part of the afternoon.

She asks about Mom's medication for depression and whether she's seen on a regular basis by a psychiatrist. I tell her that Mom had a mental health evaluation a month earlier and was judged to not be depressed and to have a mild memory impairment of about ten to twenty percent, enough to make taking care of herself difficult. I remind her that Mom also saw a psychiatrist when we were making the decision to move her to Greenway a year ago.

"If she saw another psychiatrist she'd probably just charm the doctor," I say, "making them think she's fine."

"Yes, you're probably right," she says and laughs. "I could see your mom doing that."

"Plus, her life now is really much better than it was when she lived alone, and even when she lived with me. This is a great improvement."

After a moment Daphne gently asks, "How often would you say you see your mother? Your mom told me, 'I don't remember the last time I saw Martha.'"

My breath deflates as if I've been pushed in the chest. Though I know my mother can't remember, her words still hurt. I struggle to answer Daphne without sounding defensive.

"I just saw her this past weekend. I took her to a family reunion. The weekend before that," I rattle off, growing more agitated despite my effort to conceal it, "I took her over to the cottage where she saw an old friend. We go out to lunch and dinner, to concerts, she comes over to our house for dinner, she sees her dog.

"My mother will say to me on the phone, 'It seems like so long since we talked,' when it might be just a few days since I've seen her. She just doesn't remember."

Daphne listens, then says softly, "Okay."

I'd like Mom to get out more, I think to myself, but I can't be the only one taking her out and connecting her to the world. My neighbor, Lydia, has driven across town to see Mom once or twice at Greenway, but with her children's busy home schooling schedule she can no longer visit. Daphne and I have talked before about my perhaps finding someone through a list at the Women's Resource Center of people who are available as caregivers to come and visit Mom, maybe take her out on errands or to cultural events. My only concern with this option, and the reason I haven't followed through, is safety: A paid companion would have to be extremely watchful whenever Mom is outside the flat landscape of the Greenway hallways—even walking to the parking lot is hazardous because of her slight weaving now from side to side. If Mom were with a paid companion and fell, broke a bone, a hip, a leg, her health might decline rapidly. She remains one of the more mobile residents on her floor, and I'd like to keep it that way.

"I don't know what else we might try," Daphne says. "I'll keep reminding her about activities and then I'll walk her down if she'll let me."

"I guess that's about all we can do. Thank you." I consider asking Daphne to mail me their weekly events calendar; I could call Mom and encourage her to go to the activities. It feels like too much, though, for Daphne and for me.

At the family reunion I saw for the first time not only how alone my mother looks in a crowd but how frail she seems compared to others her age. At seventy-four, Mom is relatively young to be this frail. Is her frailty caused by the tiny strokes, Alzheimer's disease, or something else?

I read in the *New York Times* that elderly people who appear to be in good health—who've had no heart attacks, major strokes or cancer—can still be disabled by frailty. Cardiovascular disease blocks circulation in the brain, other organs, and the extremities, resulting in fatigue, weakness, cognitive difficulties, and a slow walking pace. That sounds exactly like Mom.

Frailty may be avoided or delayed by exercising, maintaining healthy levels of blood pressure and cholesterol, and not smoking. When my mother lived alone she had a number of factors working against her: her two-pack-a-day habit, her sedentary lifestyle, and years of sugary junk food. And I realize now that she may have been too confused to keep track of her medication, one of which was for her high blood pressure. If her doctor had alerted me to her confusion a few years earlier, perhaps this frailty could have been prevented. Or perhaps not.

As I think of my mother's inactivity the past fifteen years, I try to imagine myself when I'm her age. I owe it to myself and my family to avoid this kind of frailty if I can. My blood pressure is fine, and aside from a puff or two in my teens I have never smoked. But at five feet six I'm nearly eighty pounds overweight. I didn't know until two years ago that I have insulin resistance and slightly high blood sugar levels, precursors to diabetes. I've now started to walk the land around our village an hour every other day; I walk two miles from my office to where I park my car downtown. I've returned to my nutritionist to monitor the amount of carbohydrates I eat and help me lose weight.

By the end of 2006, my mother has moved into Stage Five of Alzheimer's disease—moderately severe cognitive decline. (Again, I don't realize this until several years later.) As with most people in Stage Five, Mom still remembers details from her life, and she doesn't need help eating or using the toilet, but she can't remember what day it is, she needs more prompting in the shower to clean herself, and she could use more help than this assisted living facility can provide to dress appropriately. She seems to wear the same ancient pair of pants all the time—light-blue polyester pants with navy piping around the hip pockets, slightly flared at the bottom, hold-outs from the seventies. When we go outside, she doesn't remember to wear a jacket or hat, unless prompted.

On New Year's Day, I take my mother out for what I hope will be an easy lunch, nothing special. I figure I can pick Mom up at 11:30 and bring her back by 1:00. I'll coax her to sign her rent check, help her put away her Christmas gifts if she hasn't already, and be home by 2:00. I'll bring the dog so Mom can get some enjoyment out of seeing Trinka. Then, in the afternoon, I'll read and enjoy the rest of the day before returning to work the next day.

I'm fifteen minutes late arriving. I find Mom strolling out of the dining room. She leans down to love up the dog then gives me a brief hug. She's wearing the same pants, and her ancient, stained light-blue Keds, even though I gave her new, identical Keds for Christmas. Her hair still badly needs a cut; maybe she's forgotten how to walk down the hall past the auditorium to the hairdresser to schedule an appointment, as she would a year ago. It's another warning sign I've missed.

At the restaurant, Mom reaches for a packet of sugar, opens it, slowly pours it into her spoon, and eats it.

I say, "Why do you need to eat that when you are going to get dessert?"

"Because it tastes good." She opens another packet, pours it, and eats it.

After the waitress takes our order, Mom says for the third time how wonderful Trinka is. "She's such a great dog!"

"Yeah, she is." I frown, then say, "Do you feel the same way about me?" I can't help myself.

"Well, I'm not sure what to do with you today. You're a bit grumpy."

"I'm just tired," I say, but I think to myself, yes, I can be a grumpy, grumpy daughter. And that's okay sometimes. I'm allowed.

When we order dessert Mom spies the biggest sundae on the menu, with five scoops and three sauces, and says, "That's the one! I should have just had that and skipped everything else!" I worry that the other diners will look at me as if I'm taking poor care of my mother, letting her clog her narrow arteries with even more saturated fat.

I won't discover for quite some time that, for my mother's dementia, we might have more to blame on the sugar than the fat. But then, my mother's deterioration has outstripped the startling new research that implicates pre-diabetic blood sugar levels in dementia (more on this to follow).

Back inside the front entrance at Greenway, the air is thick with heat. To the right in the main sitting room two women doze in upholstered chairs, their walkers standing sentry beside them.

Upstairs, her room is also too warm. Feeling as if I could suffocate, I help her replace her old wall calendar with the new one she got for Christmas, and I encourage her to wear the new Keds. I also got her a second pair of Keds in bright pink that remind me of the red clogs she used to wear at the cottage. About the pink ones, she says now, "They're nothing I would wear. Maybe Morgan would like them." I ignore her opinion and tell her, "I bet if you wear them to dinner, you'll get lots of compliments." I realize later than Mom still has strong preferences for what she wears, that I can't shop for her as if she's a toddler.

I ask her if I can use her bathroom. On the counter by the sink I find her contact lens case with the shriveled lens inside. A year ago we picked out glasses frames but didn't buy them. She insisted at the time that she would wear her contact lens, and I didn't remind her all the time. I decide now it's time to insist on glasses and another eye exam.

I sit at her desk to write a check for her rent. Her desk is covered in old photographs—not in frames, just piles. I should put these in boxes, I think, before she dumps them in the wastebasket. A year ago when I sent her bank, which is out-of-town, a copy of my Power of Attorney and a letter requesting that I be able to sign her checks, I never heard back from them, so I continue to get Mom to sign her checks. I really should just give the bank a call, but I'm so cautious with my time I don't want to take even ten minutes to call them. It's silly, as I waste more time convincing Mom to sign each check.

When I get ready to leave, I hug Mom and kiss her on her forehead, and she hugs me back; she reaches up and gently presses my cheeks between her palms, as if to hold me still, and kisses me on the lips.

"Thank you for all your help, my dear." She keeps holding my face, and tries to look into my eyes though I want to look away.

"You're welcome, Mom. No problem."

I end my visit, as I so often do, feeling both tender toward her and eager to escape. As I close the door I glance back. She has turned toward her bed, and her thin frame, cream-colored blouse, and white hair recede into the white of her walls, the light from her window, the whiteness of her many hanging socks; with her back towards me she seems to have already forgotten that I was there.

I want to step back in, touch her shoulder, have her turn and smile at me, but I don't move. This little room with her bed with its piles of books, I think to myself, this narrow slice of space, this is her home now, her sanctuary. I know that she needs peace and quiet. I should leave her to her own life, such as it is, as much as I can. I wait a moment more. With her back still facing me she lifts a magazine from the bed and studies its cover. I pull the door shut.

Not Their Job

An eye doctor tells me that my mother must have had cataract surgery in her right eye; the implant now rests slightly askew. I vaguely remember, perhaps ten years ago, Mom telling me about the cataracts. Surgery isn't necessary, the doctor says, but glasses will make a big difference.

Mom puts on her new bifocals and I hold her arm as we walk to the car. As I drive her to lunch she keeps taking the glasses off, pushing them on top of her hair, the way she used to wear her sunglasses, like a tiara.

At Greenway, I help her pay more bills and she places the glasses on her desk. "You'll see so much better if you wear them," I say, but she leaves the glasses on the desk. Frustrated, I kiss her goodbye on the cheek. Down the hall, I ask the RAs if they could please encourage her to wear the glasses, though I doubt that they will have time to check.

I realize later that my mother is not being stubborn; she's not ignoring me because she thinks she knows best. Mom has never worn prescription glasses, only contacts. Her physical memory of glasses is that movement of pushing sunglasses up into her hair. To her, glasses belong on top of her head on a cloudy day when she's driving, on her desk when she's home. She may not be able to learn, to remember, a new habit of wearing glasses all the time.

A week later, the physician's assistant in Dr. Claiborne's office, a bearded man of about sixty, dons latex gloves and slowly strips off Mom's socks. The source of the pain in Mom's left foot is apparent: Her nicotine-yellow toenails are half an inch too long, thick and hard; some curl under. I flush, embarrassed, as if I'm a neglectful daughter who doesn't make sure that her elderly mother's toenails are properly groomed.

The PA tells me that thickened nails are a common development in the aged—caused by a fungus—and that Mom must see a podiatrist to get the nails clipped and treated.

From then on, it seems, Mom's life becomes a series of medical crises. In March, Daphne calls me to tell me that my mother's left knee and right ankle are swollen and she's having trouble walking. No one knows for sure if she fell, but I assume she rolled out of bed. Soon after she moved to Greenway, Mom began to pile magazines and books from their library on the inner edge of her bed against the wall. She seems to need more and more reading material around her because she's unable to read anything to the end. The stack extended the length of her bed and rose a foot high, with a second stack along the length of the first. She had a space only two feet wide along the outer edge of the bed on which to sleep. I pictured her scrunched up on her side, elbows and knees tucked in tight to her body. She's taken off the bed rail, the one Ben and I gave her, and stuck it in her closet.

"I don't need it," she says. I suspect that the RAs are not allowed to move residents' belongings, and that each time they change her sheets, they replace the books. A few months ago I finally ignored Mom's protests—"Just let it go; I can take care of it"—and pushed two full carts' worth back to the library. Now the pile is back.

While we wait for the results of an X-ray Mom needs to go to the bathroom but is unable to walk so I ask for a bedpan. The nurse's assistant slips it under Mom but nothing comes out. As the nurse and the nurse's assistant stand there waiting, Mom jokes that maybe she should just "twiddle" her fingers "down there" to get something to come out. I feel my cheeks redden. Mom might be making a reference to masturbation. I don't yet realize that people with dementia often make inappropriate sexual remarks. I think it's just my mother being flaky.

Because Mom can't go in the bedpan, the nurse and assistant have to help her get up, transfer her to a wheelchair, and roll her across the hallway to the bathroom. I feel like I should help, but as I've never helped Mom in the bathroom before, I'm sure I'd fumble and embarrass myself or her.

The doctor tells us that she has a sprained ligament in her knee and her ankle will be fine. She'll need a brace for her knee and a walker for a few weeks. He recommends that Mom have someone stay with her around-the-clock while her knee heals to make sure she doesn't fall down again. When I tell him that Greenway can't provide that kind of supervision he recommends hiring a private aide.

I must look distraught because he looks at me and says, "I'm so sorry. This must be very hard for you." I nod, unable to talk. I've heard so much about falls, especially broken hips, leading to nursing home placement that I fear this might be the beginning of the end for my mother. I'm completely wrung out.

I appreciate the doctor's kind words to me. It's the first time that any doctor or nurse has talked to me about my own stress. Back at Greenway the RAs let us borrow one of their walkers. A visiting nurse will help her exercise her knee. Ignoring Mom's objections, I fasten the bed rail back on her bed. At home, I look up a private home care agency in the phone book and arrange twenty-four-hour shifts. Then I retreat. I want to pace myself and delegate as much as possible. I resist making extra trips to Greenway to help Mom exercise. I expect the Greenway nurse to call me if there's a problem. I still think it's up to these other people to track her progress, not me. But am I wrong?

Mom doesn't remember that she fell; the home care agency tells me that she resists using the walker, and because she's forgotten that she hurt her knee, she can't understand why the private aides follow her around all the time. When I come to visit, an aide tells me that once, when she reminded Mom to use her walker, Mom snapped back, "Why don't *you* use it?" Understandably, by seven or eight o'clock at night, Mom gets tired of her constant companions. During the day, she enjoys chatting with them and the extra attention, but after dinner I bet her circuits overload and she just wants to be alone. When she gets testy with them, the aides tell her that, per their instructions, they must stay with her at all times. I don't think about how intrusive this must feel to my mother, how she might even feel scared.

One night the agency calls me to tell me that Mom has shoved an aide out of her room; another night they tell me she's slapped an aide. I'm disgusted, remembering that one time she slapped me on the face when I was a teenager, but the agency tells me they are used to "resistance." We decide that if Mom gets upset again, the aides will just leave the room for a few minutes and let her calm down. I'd rather cancel the aides than let her be abusive.

I find it hard not to judge my mother harshly for her behavior. I'll learn soon enough that private aides often do not receive enough training in dementia care to avoid triggering these moments of "resistance." I'll learn that, if the person with dementia grows agitated, sometimes you really do need to walk away for a few minutes, even if it means they might fall.

After three weeks Mom no longer needs the knee brace, the walker, or the private aides. Though she weaves a bit once in a while, it's the same slight weaving she's been doing for a few years.

Three blessedly uneventful months pass.

When both of my writing groups disband for the summer, my writing slips to a halt. Then, at work in mid-July, I receive a call from Greenway that precipitates a return to the pen. Sharon, the head resident assistant in Mom's section, says, "We're very concerned. Your mother has refused to eat or drink anything for twenty-four hours. She just threw up at the dining room table." She tells me that my mother also peed in her pants in the hallway. As far as I know she's never been incontinent. "She's also weaving a lot more when she walks."

I immediately drive Mom to the emergency room. She seems not to be in pain but she's pale and weak; her speech is more confused than normal, and her belly looks swollen, as if she's five months pregnant. The nurses suggest it's just constipation or dehydration; Mom should feel better after she gets some fluids, they say. They expect that, if there were a serious problem with her abdomen, she would be in pain when they palpate her stomach, but she doesn't feel anything.

I tell them, "My mother has dementia and can't remember if she felt any pain. She can only talk about what she's feeling right now, in this moment." The nurses look blankly at me. I realize that

I may know more about dementia at this point than many nurses. *More reason to stay close by*, I think to myself.

After seven hours of tests, at ten o'clock at night we find out that Mom's large intestine is obstructed. She's been refusing to eat or drink because her stomach and intestines are backed up. The young surgeon on duty tells us that as she "appears to be in no pain," the obstruction probably happened slowly, possibly caused by a tumor. The main problem, he says, is that there are a few areas in her intestine where the walls have ballooned out "to the size of a grapefruit." Her blood work shows that her white blood cell count is high, indicating that the walls are stretched thin. The danger, he tells us, is that her intestine walls could rupture, and bacteria could cause sepsis and death. He recommends immediate surgery.

My mind starts swirling. I doubt that refusing this kind of surgery was what my mother had in mind when she requested the "do not resuscitate" order in her Living Will. But I look at her pale, drawn face and the prospect of death seems almost natural. What kind of life would she return to? Days in front of a large-screen TV?

I try to calm myself, to breathe.

I ask my mother, "Do you want this surgery?"

Without hesitation she says, "Sure. I guess we'll have to!" She laughs with her usual abandon but I feel panicked, trapped.

I'm sure she's not thinking about how difficult it would be for her to recover from surgery if she forgets why she needs to lie in bed for weeks. In this moment I don't remember that, after her surgery, I could hire private aides to watch her around the clock. I acutely feel the lack of other family members, or a geriatric care manager, to call for advice.

Finally I say, "All right. Yes. Let's go ahead."

But, as we prepare for the operation, another X-ray shows that the swelling in her intestine wall has gone down. Her white blood cell count is back to normal.

"The balance is now tipping back," the surgeon explains, "toward waiting and letting her rest, rather than operating."

Thank God.

My education in geriatric medicine continues. It seems there are more obscure medical conditions than I could have imagined, and more bizarre treatments. After much ado with suctioning tubes and a colonoscopy, it turns out that Mom had a "flipped large intestine." The bottom half had flipped all the way up and the creases where it bent had twisted to form the two obstructions. It's a rare condition, and no one knows the cause. While the surgeon was in there with his probe he managed to straighten out the bowel. An X-ray shows that it's not folded up anymore, and she won't need surgery.

He tells us that once a bowel flips over it is likely to happen again, so we should watch her carefully. She can go back to Greenway the next day.

I hire the private agency again for a week to have an aide with Mom during the day at Greenway to make sure that she eats, has bowel movements, and drinks enough liquid. The nurse on Mom's floor, Brian, seems flustered, unnerved, by Mom's sudden bowel obstruction and the incident of incontinence. In the hallway he tells me, "The RAs who work here are not nurses. At night, when I'm home, they can't deal with medical problems. It's not part of their job. They don't have the training." I'm not sure what he's getting at, what he thinks I should do about all of this. I just cross my fingers and hope that Mom's large intestine doesn't flip over again.

Pressure to Move

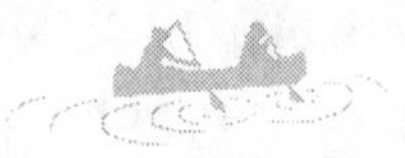

Nine days later, late on a Sunday night, an RA at Greenway calls me to tell me that Mom once again doesn't look well. They've called Brian, the nurse, at home, and the staff all think my mother should go back to the emergency room. When I arrive at Greenway a half hour later I find Mom sitting on a bench by the RA station looking pale and tired. Her stomach doesn't look bloated to me, and she's still eating and drinking, but the RAs say that she's weak and has been weaving down the halls again. I hug Mom and sit close to her, our thighs together, as if by touching her I might intuit the state of her health. Worn out, I lean over, my head in my hands, and think.

I look back up at the two RAs who stand in front of me waiting for my decision. I say, "Let's keep her here and see how she's doing in the morning. She won't get any rest in the E.R. Staying there all night would probably only make her feel worse."

They frown but say nothing.

I assume that the default setting of the Greenway staff is to send residents to the E.R. at the first sign of illness, both for the well-being of the residents and to protect the facility from lawsuits. I do feel a bit nervous ignoring their recommendation, as if I might get in trouble with the administration, but my decision feels right. I doubt Mom is in immediate danger, and she needs her sleep. To rely on my own observation and judgment rather than deferring to the staff—to say "no" to them—is a pivotal moment for me. I realize that after two years of looking out for her, I may know her better than anyone else.

The next morning the RAs tell me that my mother slept well. When I take the morning off from work to take Mom to the doctor, Dr. Claiborne finds nothing wrong with her. Mom still looks pale, so Dr. Claiborne says we should continue to make sure that she's getting enough to drink. I'll keep the private aides during the day.

At the end of July, Ben and the kids and I go away for a week's vacation in the Adirondack Mountains. Looking back, I can't believe I did this, but I leave my cell phone at home. It's true that it's my first cell phone and I'm not used to carrying it all the time, but I also crave a total break away from worrying about Mom's health. I need a vacation, and I feel that Ben and our children deserve my time and attention. I deliberately make myself unavailable. For some reason, I never imagine that while we are away for a few days Mom might be back in the hospital. And I naively expect that if there are any problems, it would be Greenway's responsibility to handle them. The part of me that's still getting used to being responsible for my mother resists being on call all the time, resists being the adult.

When we return on a Saturday evening I find messages on our answering machine and on my cell phone from Daphne,

Greenway's case manager, saying that they called an ambulance to take Mom to the hospital because she wasn't eating or drinking again and she looked "six months pregnant." I flush, pierced with guilt. When I call them I apologize to an RA for being out of touch, aware of how lame I must sound. She tells me that my mother went to the hospital five days ago and returned three days ago. An X-ray showed that, sure enough, her bowels twisted again, but with fluids the kinks worked themselves out and she's fine now, she "looks good."

When I see Mom the next day she looks great—lots of color in her face, lots of energy—but I can't stop thinking of her alone, curled under a white blanket in the E.R. I pray that she doesn't remember. I give her a long hug, and from that moment on, remain on guard for the next call.

Ever since my mother's first bowel obstruction, she's been incontinent. When she sleeps at night and naps during the day, she soaks the sheets and her clothes. Several times a day the RAs have to change her bed, wipe her down, get her dressed again. I know nothing about incontinence and trust that Greenway will do what they need to do to keep her clean and dry. I do wonder if Mom's progressed into a later stage of dementia. Does her brain no longer register the pressure of a full bladder? The urine either leaks out when she's awake or gushes out when she falls asleep.

In mid-August, when I swing by for a visit, Brian, the nurse, stops me in the hallway. "With all of your mom's health issues all of a sudden, I wonder if maybe she's had a small stroke."

I say, "Her doctor thinks it might be a side effect of one of her medications." A few weeks ago, after I kept asking Dr. Claiborne about trying one of the medications to lessen the symptoms of Alzheimer's disease, she agreed to start my mother on one of them, a popular brand. We weren't sure it would help at this point, but we felt it couldn't hurt to try.

Brian shakes his head. "Her doctor has no clue what's wrong with your mom."

The nurse may be right, but even though I know Mom had small strokes when she lived alone, I can't wrap my mind around the word "stroke" right now, standing in a hallway. If Brian had sat down with me in his office and explained his concerns more slowly I might have let the word penetrate. Instead, I focus on the new drug, and wonder as well if Mom has just moved on to a more serious phase of dementia.

Later that day when I call Daphne, she tells me that my mother is now in a "gray area"; with the incontinence the Greenway staff may not be able to manage all of Mom's care. According to our state's regulations for assisted living, and the employee contracts for this facility, RAs may give my mother a shower only every other morning, and they may supervise her dressing herself, but not every day. They cannot physically help her dress, or pull her Depends on or off. The RAs can check on Mom several times a day and twice in the night, and change her bedclothes if they get wet. I assume that Mom can deal with dressing and the Depends on her own, with supervision and prompting.

Daphne never comes out and says clearly that if Mom does not get outside help she cannot continue to live there, but it's implied. I offer to hire a private aide to come in for an hour or two on the alternate mornings Greenway cannot give Mom a shower, and every day for an hour in the afternoon to make sure Mom is not walking around in wet pants, as the staff reports she has been. I hesitate to add more hours of private aides because of the cost to Mom's savings account, but it can't be helped. Daphne and I agree that this plan might work. She suggests I call a woman named Maggie who works with other residents at Greenway; while she's already in the building Maggie could stop by and check on Mom. And she's less expensive than the other agency.

I trust that if there are any problems, the RAs will report them to Brian or to Daphne, and that Brian or Daphne will, in turn, report them to me. I have perhaps too much faith in their channels of communication.

At a check-up, Dr. Claiborne takes Mom off the Alzheimer's medication. We doubt the medication has any connection with my mother's sudden problems, but we eliminate it anyway. We don't talk about the possibility that she may have had a small stroke.

A week after Maggie starts helping my mother I get a call from Daphne.

"I've met with the staff, we've discussed your mom, and we all think that it may be time for her to be evaluated for nursing home placement."

The thought saddens me deeply. I don't want my mother in a nursing home so soon. She's still mobile and talkative and just too "with it." But I trust Greenway's opinion because they know more than I do about such transitions. Daphne says that a nurse from the county's Long-term Care Services office will conduct a medical evaluation called a Patient Review Instrument (PRI). Greenway's main concerns are her recurring bowel obstructions, which they believe may need round-the-clock nursing care to monitor, and the incontinence. I tell Daphne, "I don't want to see my mother in a nursing home just because of incontinence, but I'm willing to cooperate with whatever you and Long-term Care recommend."

The PRI nurse meets with me and my mother in Mom's room. I explain to Mom that the woman is a visiting nurse who's going to ask a few questions "just to see how you're doing." I never mention the possibility of a nursing home. The nurse quietly and patiently determines that Mom is actually doing quite well except for needing some extra help to stay clean and dry. "The bowel inversions may not continue," she says, "and if they do, they are not the kind of condition that should require more than a short visit to the hospital." Mom looks good, she's coherent and talkative, she's strong, and she walks well without a walker with minor weaving only when she's particularly tired or dehydrated. The nurse tells me that she will take the answers to our questions with her and determine Mom's "score" tomorrow, but it seems clear to her, she tells me in the hallway, that my mother does not need a nursing home at this time. What she needs is what she is getting now with Maggie—extra help pulling the Depends on and off, staying in dry clothes, and getting her bed linens changed if the Depends leak.

I excuse myself from Mom for a moment and walk with the PRI nurse down the hall to talk with her and Brian. In Brian's office I'm annoyed, Brian's defensive, the discussion tense. Brian says, "I never suggested in the staff meeting that your mom needed a nursing home."

I say, "I hear one thing from you and the opposite from Daphne. Who should I go to when I need information?"

He takes a deep breath in and out through his nostrils. "It's supposed to be Daphne's job to pass on the opinions of the staff."

The PRI nurse watches us and says nothing. Still confused, I walk the PRI nurse to the entrance. "I'm sorry about that," I say.

She smiles. "I understand. In fact, I try to listen really hard to what family members think." She looks at me for a long moment, then says, "I'm often called to do an evaluation for a nursing home when it turns out the person's really not ready for one." She smiles again, studies my eyes, then touches my arm. "Good luck."

This moment in the parking lot is the first time I suspect that I might feel less stress if my mother lived elsewhere. Perhaps some of this confusion could be preventable.

But I don't know where else to take Mom. I'd forgotten about Maple Grove, the assisted living facility with the "memory care" cottage for people with dementia that two years ago I shied away from visiting. I assume that my mother still doesn't need that kind of dementia residence, just as she's still not ready for a nursing home. In my mind, she has no place to go.

Part III

REHAB

Fractured

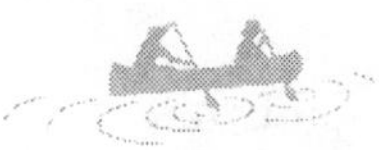

In mid-August, Sharon, the head RA, calls me at work. "Shit," I say under my voice when our assistant tells me that Greenway is on the phone. I've learned that calls from them, infrequent as they are, can only mean bad news.

"Hi, Martha," Sharon says in a concerned voice. "Your mom seems to be in a lot of pain. She can't put any weight on her right leg, and she can't walk. We don't know what happened but we think she should go to the hospital." At Greenway I find Mom waiting for me in a wheelchair inside the front entrance with another resident keeping her company.

"There she is!" Mom cries out when she sees me and gives me a big smile. While she normally sits and walks perfectly erect—a resident once asked me if she used to be a model—now in the wheelchair she's hunched over, one shoulder twisted down toward the arm of the chair, the collar of her pink cardigan bunched sideways.

When I reach down to give her a hug, Mom doesn't pull me close as she usually does; she places her hands gingerly on my shoulders, then releases her hands and pats her palms in the air above her thighs.

"I've got something...going on...down here," she says, pausing twice in the middle of the sentence to find the right words. This hesitation started a month earlier with the first bowel inversion and the sudden incontinence, and seems to be another clue that she probably had a small stroke, but I don't make the connection for many months.

"I know, Mom. I'm here to take you to the hospital."

As the medics wheel my mother toward the door she points back to me. "This is my daughter," she tells them. "She's the one who knows."

Mom's vitals are fine, and an EKG, to rule out a fall caused by a heart attack, is also normal. I call Maggie on my cell phone to see if she can give me more information about what happened. She tells me that when she arrived at Greenway this morning she found Mom half in, half out of her bed, kneeling on the floor with the rest of her body leaning over the bed "as if she was praying." Maggie was able to get her up and help her take a shower and get dressed, but after an hour Mom started to complain of searing pain in her leg.

An hour later a doctor tells Mom that her pelvis is fractured near her groin. She doesn't need surgery, but it will take several weeks to heal.

"Where, exactly, is her pelvis?" I ask the doctor, feeling a bit foolish. He invites me to come out into the center of the nursing station and look at the X-ray. I stand behind him as he sits in front of a large computer screen on which appears the ghostly outline of my mother's hips. I've never seen an X-ray of my mother's body. The intimacy makes me feel an even stronger calling to protect her. The doctor points out two narrow, symmetrical strips of bone between her legs near her crotch. On each side a faint but jagged line stitches into the bone. "It hurts when she moves her legs," he says, "because the fractured bone is connected to the muscle tissue." I wince.

When I have to leave, who will remind her to lie still? Who will believe her when she says it hurts? She can't afford a private aide to sit with her around the clock until this heals. At least if Mom tries to get up, the pain may dissuade her from trying again.

Mom is admitted to a room on the third floor, and the doctor on rounds comes in with the nurse to give Mom a quick exam. They ask her to lift her legs, flex her ankles and wiggle her toes. They are sometimes careful and sometimes too quick. When they leave, I reach to gently squeeze her hand.

"Are you all right?"

"No." She stares straight ahead at the foot of her bed. "They think I've done something wrong, and they're blaming me."

At 8:30 I tell her that I have to head home.

She smiles. "Do what you need to do for you," she says, one of her old 12-step sayings.

My mother is incredibly selfless, I think. Later I realize that she'd probably already forgotten where she was and why, and considered my goodbye the end of a normal visit.

It's a late Saturday afternoon and I'm visiting Mom at the hospital after spending the entire day cleaning the cottage with Ben. We've begun to rent it out each week of the summer that we can't use it. We've bought all new furniture, repaired the broken concrete steps, cleaned the roof and chimney, and purchased new dishware, towels and linens. The cottage is cozy and beautiful again, our renters love it, and we are fully booked. We're not able to save much rental income, though, as the refurbishing, repair and maintenance are expensive, the property taxes high. Renting the cottage simply allows us to keep it.

Mom has been moved to a new room, and I find her in a double room in the bed farthest from the window, with her bare feet and legs sticking out from her blanket. My first thought is that she's spilled some tea. I ring for a hospital aide to change her sheets. Two aides come and tell me that Mom's been incontinent, which catches me by surprise for some reason, maybe because I've never seen her wet. They roll Mom first onto one side and then the other so they can slip clean sheets and a pad under her. Mom cries out when she has to move her hips. Though I've never seen her in so much pain, all I think I can do is stand by, passive; I assume the aides know what they're doing. But afterwards I wonder if I'm wrong. How often do they read the patients' charts?

As usual I've brought treats, today a single serving packet of Oreos from the hospital cafeteria and a pint of sweet Bing cherries from the farm stand down the road. As she eats, I sit in the chair at the foot of her bed and read the local paper. Three hours later, I kiss her goodbye, as we always do now, on the lips. I smooth her hair and lightly sweep my hands in a crescent around her face.

"Oh, I like that!" She gives me a bright smile as I move away from the bed. "I love you," she says.

"I love you, too."

The next day, Sunday, is my secular Sabbath, the one day a week I try to do no work and just enjoy the quiet blessings of life. I wake up not wanting to go anywhere, and rest all morning in the living room, reading. Certainly a hospital visit can be a blessing, but I still see such visits as duty, not pleasure.

By noon, though, I realize I need to call Maggie, the private aide, to tell her that Mom's in the hospital and won't be back at Greenway for a while. Maggie takes this opportunity to tell me that, at Greenway, Mom was not receiving a shower in between her visits. "I would find your mom wearing the same clothes, the same underwear, I left her in two days before. Sometimes her underwear was wet."

I tell her that Mom was probably resisting being changed for bed, and sleeping in her clothes. But the Greenway staff could have insisted that Mom change on the alternate days that Maggie was not there.

"I really recommend Maple Grove," Maggie says, referring to the other assisted living place in town, the one with the dementia cottage.

I thank her for telling me, and say I'll think about it.

After lunch my guilt about leaving Mom alone in the hospital pushes aside my inertia and I drive the five minutes there. As I leave the house Morgan asks me to wait while she picks a red pear from our tree for Grammy. I bring as well a heavy vase and pick fresh flowers for her from my garden: snapdragons in maroon, orange, and white; matching strawflowers in the colors of an October sunset. At a convenience store down the hill I pick up the Sunday *Times* for myself, and a small packet of peanut M&M's for Mom. Mom used to love peanut M&M's when she stopped drinking; at that time her local 12-step group encouraged eating sugary things as a substitute for alcohol.

I find Mom sitting up in her hospital bed but slumped a bit, staring off into space.

"I wondered where you were," she says. A glint in her eye quickly fades.

We find a movie on the TV with Cary Grant and Humphrey Bogart. Though she can't remember their names, Mom seems to recognize their voices. We continue to click and find the movie *Anna and the King* with Jodie Foster and Chow Yun Fat. I ask Mom if she remembers when I was in the musical *The King and I* in sixth grade and she says no. I remind her that I played the oldest of the children in the processional march. I had to wait to hear the music begin—dah, dum-dum, dummm—and then lead the line of children out onto the stage. I tell her I had to wear short, billowing pants that looked like giant diapers and that we all had our hair dyed black and pulled up in buns. She finds this amusing. I tell her that I got to sing on stage with the other children in Anna's class. Now, as I sit next to Mom, I reach for her hand, sit back, and sing "Getting to Know You." Mom knows the first few lines and sings along. I'm self-conscious at first, nervous about what Mom's roommate on the other side of the curtain might think, or what the staff will think if they can hear us. But singing together with Mom, stroking her hand, this worry passes, and, for a few moments, all is "bright and breezy."

After an hour and a half with my mother I tell her I need to go home. On the back of her lunch menu I write her a note in big block letters:

Mom,

Do not get out of bed! If you need something, call the nurse by pressing the red button on the TV remote.

You have a fractured pelvis, and it needs to heal!

Love, Martha

First thing Monday morning, from work, I call the hospital's discharge nurse. Mom must leave the hospital and spend a few weeks in a rehabilitation center.

"What would you prefer to do?" she asks me. "Greenway cannot take her back."

I tell her that I've heard good things about the rehab center at a nursing home called Lakebridge. But I'm not sure how I'm going to transport my mother if she's in too much pain to get into my car.

"People sometimes hire a wheelchair ambulance," she says. "But why don't we worry about crossing that bridge when we get to it?" She's cheerfully dismissive.

I want to tell her, but I don't, that I've already missed many days of work taking Mom back and forth to the hospital, and I'd prefer to be able to plan ahead, to not be surprised by a call one morning that she's ready to be discharged.

After work I swing home to pick up Morgan, who wants to come with me to the hospital this time, maybe just to spend more time with me, as I've been so distracted lately. When we arrive we find Mom standing up next to her bed as if about to walk off.

"Oh, I was just coming to see you!" She smiles at us, but doesn't greet Morgan by name.

She's unhooked the alarm that is supposed to alert the nurses if she tries to get out of bed. Usually a string connects a small clip on the shoulder of her hospital gown to a magnetic hook on a black box the size of a deck of cards strapped with Velcro to the bed railing. If she moves too far off the bed the magnetic hook is pulled off the black box and a loud alarm goes off. I see that the clip, string, and black box are not only unattached, but neatly coiled up on the tray next to her bed. Wily and persistent, Mom's figured out how to remove the whole alarm system intact. The aides and nurses down the hall are none the wiser.

The only other way to keep her on bed rest would be to strap her down or to drug her, neither of which the hospital wants to do. Of course I wouldn't want to see her out of it on drugs or tied down, but I worry that she will fall again and hurt herself even worse. It still does not occur to me that I could hire a private aide for the daytime hours; I assume it's the hospital's job to keep her safe.

Two aides help Mom into bed, and with the head of the bed raised up, she sits and digs into the cheesecake with strawberry sauce I brought. Morgan has chocolate cake and they trade bites. As I watch Mom enjoy her cheesecake I think of how this is like parenting a three-year-old: as long as she has something she can give all of her attention to, even a small thing like a snack, she is happy and life is good. I can sit quietly and just be with her; I don't need to make conversation. Morgan watches a children's station on the TV. I smile at Mom while she chats about things that I can't really make sense of. Once again I slip down the hall to pilfer a *Time*, a *Woman's Day*, a *Vogue*. Mom glances at the covers of the magazines but tosses them to the foot of the bed.

"Now, clean up after yourself," she says.

"But," I say, annoyance flashing through my veins, "I got those for you to read when you're bored."

"Oh—okay." She laughs.

In a moment she says, "When are we leaving?"

"Morgan and I will leave soon," I tell her, "but you have to stay in bed here and rest. You have a fracture that needs to heal."

"I do?"

I look around for the green piece of paper on which I wrote the letter to her yesterday but it's been thrown away. When I write her another one I wish I had tape so I could fasten it to something that won't get tossed. Mom reads it over and over; each time is a revelation.

I fill out the nursing home application form for rehabilitation, then rise to leave. Mom's eyes are bright and she leans forward. "So, you're taking me with you?"

"No, Mom, I'm just taking Morgan home. I'll be back tomorrow."

"So when…can I…expect you?"

I tell her I'll be there after work, around 3:00. I remind Mom again to not get out of bed without help and the woman in the other bed calls out to me, "I'll keep an eye on her! If she gets out of bed I'll tell her to get back in!" I peek around the curtain and give Mom's roommate a big thank you, but I feel too drained to appreciate this angel helping me watch over my mother. Mom laughs.

I have my other angels. Maggie is warm and thoughtful enough to forewarn me, discreetly, that I am choosing the wrong rehab center. When I tell Maggie that I've asked that Mom go to Lakebridge for rehab I can hear her inhale sharply.

"I wouldn't want to see her there." She hesitates as if it would be unprofessional for her to criticize the place.

I agree to check out a different place she recommends, but time is running out—quickly.

On Wednesday, Morgan and I arrive at the hospital to find my mother swaddled in an adult diaper, flat on her back looking up at the ceiling. Her thin legs lie uncovered; her feet are bare, her brown hospital-issued socks strewn at the foot of the bed. With her body curved toward the edge of the bed, her head rests only three-quarters of the way up, as if she got out of bed and only made it back in half way. The Depends lie loose and baggy around her hips. The tabs stick out. I feel a twinge of anger at the hospital for leaving her like this, but mostly I feel numb.

Mom looks up at me with a small, embarrassed smile, as if she's trying to lighten a depressing situation. "This is...new...for me."

I swallow hard and reach for her hand. "You mean wearing Depends?"

"Yes," she says, "these...diapers."

I take a breath, keep looking down into her eyes, and try to explain.

"Sometimes you're incontinent, Mom. You leak urine. It's fine. It happens to a lot of older people." I grope for something else to say to reassure her. "Lots of people wear these Depends under their clothes and you don't even know it. Probably the hospital put these on you so you won't be sitting in a wet bed."

Mom listens, and with her usual trust in me seems a bit less embarrassed. "If you say so, sweetie."

It smells in her room, and I notice a wastebasket next to Mom's bed full of rolled-up wet diapers. Why should she have to lie right next to that? I move the wastebasket into the bathroom.

"Mom, I bet you'll be glad to know that you'll be out of here soon—maybe even tomorrow. You'll be going to a rehabilitation center so your pelvic fracture can heal." Woodside called me today and said they had a bed. I try to avoid using the words "nursing home," but refer to it as rehab. "It'll just be temporary," I say. For the next ten minutes I explain several times why she needs rehab.

"I want to know more," she says.

Without realizing it I find myself trying to distract Mom, much as I would a preschooler. On the bedside table I spot the two photo albums that I'd brought in another day.

"Did you have a chance to look at these?" Oh, yes, she says. I place the album with photos of the cottage on the bed next to her lap. With her thin but strong arms Mom holds the album upright on her hips without a sign of pain. She brightens as soon as she opens it to the first page.

"I see you," she says, pointing to herself in a photo, "but who is this little one?"

"That's me, Mom." My stomach contracts. "And that's you, when you were a bit younger than I am now." I point to her face in the photo with the black cat-eye sunglasses.

Silent, Mom shakes her head as if in disbelief.

"You know, Mom, two years ago you helped me label all these photos."

"I did?"

In the evening, I tell Ben about my afternoon with Mom, and he gives me a long hug and a kiss. He often uses humor to try to lighten my mood, and now he smiles and reminds me of our standing joke. "Remember," he says, "if one of us ever gets dementia, we're going to borrow a gun, go out into the woods, and have ourselves a little hunting accident." I laugh, but in this moment it sounds like a darn good plan. Messy, but definite.

Very early the next morning, a Thursday, the hospital discharge nurse calls to tell me without warning that Mom needs to leave that day. I agree to a 12:30 discharge so I can get at least a couple of hours of work done in the morning. I tell the discharge nurse to let her go on her own with the ambulance; I will meet Mom at Woodside. I still think that professionals like nurses and an ambulance crew should be able to keep a person with dementia calm and unafraid. I still try to delegate as much as possible.

But only five minutes after I hang up, as I rinse the breakfast dishes, I turn the faucet off and sigh. I can't let Mom leave the hospital and arrive at a new place without a family member by her side. I need to be there to explain to her what's going on, to talk to her. This may be the first time I accept that my mother's comfort is more important than my convenience.

Chunks of Life

Woodside is a two-story extension of a four-floor nursing home, its white, cement buildings flanked by a courtyard of small trees, flower gardens, and a blue picket fence. Inside, four staff members sit bent over paperwork at the front desk. When the medics wheel Mom into the lobby, the staff members all look up at the same time and greet us with a cheer of "Welcome!" I'm used to being invisible at the hospital so I feel a bit embarrassed by the attention. I force a smile. Mom, of course, beams.

There's something antiseptic permeating the air, minty and solid: unnatural, but not quite unpleasant. I'm pleased to learn that Mom will have a bed by the window. The large room with two beds and a curtain down the middle feels more homelike than I expected, with walls painted in light green, paisley drapes tied back on the large window, and a matching wallpaper border along the ceiling.

I see that her roommate is a woman perhaps in her nineties wearing a hospital gown and tucked into bed under what looks like a handmade afghan. This is the woman the director told me would be heading home the next day. I'm so focused on my mother I don't think to say hello. The woman is silent but follows us with her eyes.

The floor supervisor, Peggy, stops by to introduce herself, then Mom and I sit and look at her new space. Between the slats of the window blinds we can see a leafy side street lined with clapboard houses. The registered nurse, Sarah, arrives and squats in front of Mom's chair so that she's looking up at Mom when she asks the usual questions: How did you fall? Are you in any pain? I try to catch her eye to tell her that Mom isn't able to remember her accident, that her answers may sound probable but won't be accurate. Sarah nods in my direction but doesn't return my look or try to include me in the conversation. She speaks to me only when she stands up. "I'm happy to talk to you if you have any questions," she says. "Just give me a call."

A call? I think to myself. You'll listen to me on the phone, but not now, in person?

When Sarah leaves I notice that my mother's roommate has a large mug of water with a straw, but Mom doesn't. In the hallway by the vending machines I see Peggy, the floor supervisor, again. She tells me that she will rig my mother's bed with a hidden alarm: under her sheet an alarm pad will sound if she takes her weight off of the bed.

"I think your mom might be a 'fiddler,'" she says with a smile. "If we attach the alarm to her shirt she'll just unhook it."

"You're right," I say, deeply relieved that Peggy is so observant, that she has already noticed this tic of my mother's and come up with a way to try to keep her safe.

When I return to Mom's room the social worker, Katherine, stops by, accompanied by the physical therapist, Abby. They are both warm and upbeat women in their forties, with short hair and dangly earrings, and wearing Birkenstocks. They introduce themselves and ask for my name. They ask Mom to smile for a photo—"so we can be sure to give you the right medicine," they tell her. To get Mom to smile, Abby makes moose antlers with her hands behind Katherine's head, and Mom laughs and makes moose antlers, too.

Abby, the physical therapist, squats down in front of Mom's chair as the nurse did, and asks Mom a familiar round of questions. Again I try to catch her eye, and, failing that, pipe up and tell her that Mom won't remember and that her answers won't be too accurate. I worry that if they get the wrong information they might ask her to do things she shouldn't be doing and she may fall again or strain her injury. Later I realize that by asking her all these questions the staff is probably just trying to assess her memory for themselves.

Abby helps Mom put on her Keds. "These must be new!" Abby says and looks up at me. I appreciate her smile as a way to acknowledge my care for my mother. She gets Mom to her feet. "Judy, I need you to walk with me. We're going to go down the hallway so we can weigh you." I stay in the room to fill out the paperwork.

Ten minutes later Abby comes back for me—"Martha, I need your help," she says calmly.

In the hallway I can see that Mom has planted herself in a chair. She's refused to walk the remaining twenty feet back to her room. She wears that exasperated "I've had enough" expression I know so well: her eyes are closed and her lips are pursed. She's tilted her head back against the chair, each arm balanced on an armrest, each hand draped over the end, bent at the wrist, regal.

"Judy, Martha's here to help you walk back to your room."

No response.

"Will you let her help you?"

Silence, then with a sigh Mom says to Abby, "Yes, but only if you go away. Leave me alone and stop yapping at me."

"It's just a few more feet," Abby says.

"Shut up."

Abby turns to me. "Your mom was even nastier to me a few minutes ago." Her tone is matter-of-fact, not accusatory.

For a long minute Abby and I stand and wait. Finally Mom pushes herself out of the chair, holds onto the walker, and continues shuffling up the hallway. She stops after a few steps. "It hurts," she cries, and points to the back of her right leg. Her eyes well up.

"You can make it, Judy." Abby seems so confident that I try not to worry and instead do what I can to encourage Mom to make it back to her bed. I walk ahead of her, looking back. "Here's your room; it's not much farther."

When she finally reaches her bed, Mom says to Abby, "Go away." She leans back onto the bed, her legs half off, and looks up at the ceiling. Abby takes a few steps back, silent.

"It's okay, Mom. You're almost done. Will you let us help you get all the way on the bed?"

"Fine."

Once Mom's curled up on her side, Abby asks to speak to me in the hallway.

"I don't want you to feel bad," she says. "We know she has dementia, and that she's not always going to remember things. We're used to that. And we're also used to people resisting and saying mean things to us. She might be sun-downing," she says, referring to a common symptom of dementia, an increase in irritability in the late afternoon and evening.

"She did walk a long way, farther than she wanted to. But it was good for me to see what her limit is. Next time we won't go so far."

All I can think to say is "Okay." I feel powerless to protect my mother, bewildered, and sad.

After Abby leaves, I sit and hold Mom's hand. I press gently, as if to absorb and lighten her pain. She falls into a thin sleep. I turn to the pile of paperwork to fill out the usual forms—social history, events leading to injury, burial fund, cognitive status, places of residence, consent to release, Designated Representative Agreement—and my own tears start to fall.

Before dinner this first night, an aide helps Mom into a wheelchair, then brushes her hair, which delights her. I realize I've never brushed my mother's hair. It seems so intimate.

The dining room is Spartan compared to the fancy, chandeliered dining room at Greenway: blank white walls, the wooden tables bare except for red paper placemats and tiny plastic glasses. We both notice that there is some sort of garden patio outside—I can see cleomes and black-eyed Susans—but the door says "Not an Exit." Waiting to be served, people stare off into space or nap like birds with their chins tucked into their chests.

We sit and wait for what feels like forever, maybe twenty minutes, while the aides wheel in the rest of the patients. Some patients walk in on their own, as does a woman of about ninety who shuffles in with a walker and sits across from us at our table.

"Are you new here?" she asks my mother.

"Yes, I guess so. I just got...established...a while ago."

The woman pulls on a green sweater. "You ask them to turn the air conditioning down and they say they can't; only the maintenance men can do it."

"Are you cold, Mom, in your short-sleeved shirt?"

"Yes, a bit."

"I'll be right back." From the car I retrieve the sweater we left in another bag.

When I come back Mom announces to the room, "This is my daughter!"

When she finally gets her dinner, Mom ignores the turkey salad and potato salad and heads right for the cupcake. As it's on her plate, she seems to assume that she must use a knife and fork, and proceeds to cut the cupcake into pieces, which she gingerly lifts to her mouth with the fork. She wipes the crumbs off the side of her knife onto the crest of her turkey salad. She shovels up the pieces of cupcake liner with her fork and deposits them in the valley between the twin mounds of protein and starch as if the whole plate and everything on it is just a background landscape for the sweet dessert. I shake my head in disbelief.

"You should probably eat your whole dinner, not just the dessert."

"Am I going to tell *you* what to eat?" she retorts.

"Fair enough." I am being obnoxious, and I wouldn't want someone telling me what I should eat—but I can't help myself. Mom doesn't seem to register feelings of hunger, just as she doesn't seem to feel mild pain or the need to urinate. Is this another glitch in her brain?

I grow tired of sitting with Mom at the dinner table, but it never occurs to me to roll her back to her room myself. I assume she has to wait for the aides.

"I have to go finish some paperwork, Mom. I'll see you in a few minutes." I don't worry that she'll feel scared or alone because she seems too out-of-it to even know where she is.

Five minutes later, Mom appears outside the door of her room, alone, propelled in her wheelchair by her blue-socked feet.

"There you are!" She taps her heels on the floor to come to a stop, and reaches her arms out to me.

"You made it back on your own!" I say. I can't believe she remembered how to go from the dining room to her new room.

"I didn't know where you were!" Her eyes are huge, like those of a young child who has lost her mother in a department store.

A wave of guilt flashes through me as if I were that mother, too engrossed in her shopping list, in too much of a hurry to get home, to notice that she's left her child alone in another aisle.

I drop the paperwork on the bed and step out in the hallway to hug her. From around the corner Peggy, the floor supervisor, appears, erect and calm. She smiles and winks at me, then leans down in front of Mom's wheelchair to loop something white that looks like a wristband around Mom's right ankle. It has a small white box attached to it.

"This is an alarm," she explains to me. "Your mom announced to the aides back there that she was going to go outside and find you and your car. If she does try to go out the door, this alarm will automatically lock the doors." She doesn't offer an explanation directly to Mom besides a simple "We're going to put this around your ankle, okay Judy?"—but that seems fine to Mom as she pays little attention to this new appendage. I feel jittery, though, with the realization that Mom missed me so much that she tried to find me outside. Impressed that she remembered that I had a car parked outside. That there even was an outside.

By seven o'clock I'm ready to go. I help Mom out of her wheelchair and into the wingback chair by the bed. I've watched the aides enough times that I don't need to ring for help; I ask her to push herself up out of the wheelchair, stand, then pivot around to the chair using the walker for support. Feeling a need to nest her space before I leave, I move the bedside table closer to the head of her bed. That way, the phone and the magazines are within her reach when she sits in bed. I place a few magazines on the foot of her bed ("There, something for you to read," I say). I clip the buzzer for the aides onto her sweater. I trot to the main desk to ask for a remote for Mom's TV. Back in her room I feel I can't leave Mom alone without some sort of way for her to remember why she's there. On the back of a scrap of paper I write another letter:

Dear Mom,

This is Woodside Rehabilitation Center. You will be here a few weeks until the fracture in your pelvis heals. Then you will go back to your own room at Greenway. Try to cooperate with the physical therapist. It may hurt, but you have to exercise.

If you need to get up or go to the bathroom, press the white button clipped to your shirt. Do not get up on your own.

I will see you tomorrow.

Love, Martha

I lean over Mom's chair and look down into her eyes.

"It's getting pretty late, Mom. I need to go home and see my family—Ben and the kids."

Immediately her eyes well up with tears. "I need to see my family, too."

"I know, Mom." I am your family, I think to myself, and I'll be here, every day.

"I'll see you tomorrow, and maybe on Saturday I can bring Ben and Andrew and Morgan."

Her eyes still lock on mine. She lifts her chin and smiles.

"Do what you need to do for you," she says.

At home in the kitchen Ben pulls me close—"I'm sorry, honey"—and fixes me dinner. I tell him about my day, but realize that most of my caregiving duties for my mother are invisible to him. They happen away from him, out of sight.

I check my email for the cottage rental business (potential renters like to hear back from me within twenty-four hours), then pull on my swimsuit and walk down to the pond. It's almost completely dark, the full moon partly hidden by mist, the air still pressing its heat to my face and shoulders. Birds swoop in wide arcs over my head, toads croak from the cattails, and out in the deep end, a fish jumps.

I think of how my mother used to love to swim, not in ponds so much but in Silver Lake, and in our secret swimming hole in the Adirondack woods. At the lake, Mom would always doggie-paddle back and forth in front of the shale beach, careful to keep her hair and contact lens out of the water, buoyed under her chest by a red, square cushion from the boathouse. As I sidestroke through the pond I imagine that I am swimming for my mother, taking her place. With Mom in a nursing home rehab center, I truly feel as if she is no longer in this world.

Though I find it hard now to picture anything other than her decline, I force myself to stop thinking that way. Before her injury, only two weeks earlier, I convinced her to try the new wooden swing at the cottage and she enjoyed being pushed back and forth.

Just let it all go, I tell myself—Mom swimming or not swimming, or eating only a cupcake for dinner. I should take my cue from my mother. If she doesn't care about swimming any more, I shouldn't feel sorry for her when I think of her no longer doing it. If she chooses to eat just sweets for one meal, I shouldn't worry that she'll go hungry.

That night I can't get to sleep for several hours. Then, in the middle of the night, I wake up, my heart racing, from a nightmare. I dreamt I'm standing next to an open window on the third or fourth floor of a brick apartment building. Outside the window I can see an airshaft in the center of the building, nothing but brick walls on all sides, a few windows, and a tiny square of cement courtyard below. Cupped in my hands I hold a tiny puppy, a soft, floppy Lab with brown eyes. I drop the puppy out the window. I can see that the dog is still alive, writhing on the cement. It looks up at me with its big eyes, silent. I want to rush down and help it but there's no way to get there, no door to the courtyard. I turn my head and avert my eyes.

* * *

The next day, after work, I stop by and roll Mom to the courtyard. At a round table under a low-slung tree, we sip cups of water and enjoy the shade, the red geraniums, and the occasional breeze parting the late-August heat.

"That feels good," Mom says.

Abby hustles by, and smiles and waves at Mom as she passes our table.

"Why…the wave?" Mom calls out.

"Because I saw you smiling at me!" Abby says, turning back to stand beside Mom. Abby looks at me. "You have the same smile!"

I give her a reluctant half-smile, still thinking of how hard she'd pushed my mother the day before.

Turning back to Mom she says, "You did great today, Judy."

As Abby starts to walk away, Mom calls out to her again. "Give me a good… report…for the day!"

"A-plus, Judy," Abby calls back. "You definitely get an A-plus!"

The next day, a Saturday, I'm more than ready for a break. I have visited Mom every day since she went to the hospital with the pelvic fracture. Since Ben and Morgan are going downtown to the library, and the rehab center lies on the way, I ask them to stop in and see Mom for a short visit. I'll feel less guilty about skipping a day if someone else sees her. And if Ben stops to see her, he might have a clearer understanding of what I've been dealing with every day.

It turns out that Ben and Morgan spend more time with Mom than I expect they will. Ben buys Mom a small chocolate bar from the vending machine in the staff lounge, then wheels her outside to the courtyard. Morgan tells me later that her dad smiled the whole time. I'm surprised, and I love him dearly for doing this willingly, considering how he feels about her.

• • •

Sunday, I stop to see Mom in the late afternoon after cleaning the cottage. I am still grimy, in a frayed shirt, my greasy hair in a ponytail and with a sheen of sweat on my face.

"Oh, was that good for you?" she asks, meaning the cleaning, I think.

"Sure," I say. "I like to see the cottage nice and clean."

I tell her the lake was a gorgeous deep blue today, with huge waves and whitecaps.

"Was it…did…the lake…suffice?" she asks.

"Sure," I say again, though I'm not positive I know what she's asking. Was the lake beautiful in its own right? Did I feel happy there? Yes.

I tell her that the neighbors right next to us were there for the weekend. Mom gives me a blank look. They were in the brown and white cottage, I explain. "Charlie Smith's place."

She lights up at his name. "Oh, sure!" she says.

"His youngest sister owns the cottage now. Charlie's ninety-one and in a nursing home."

Mom looks sad. As she tries to find the right words to express how she feels she tilts her head and smiles at me as if she's amused at herself. She raises her hands in front of her chest, her palms facing each other a foot apart, and packs the air between them as if creating a large snowball.

"I'd forgotten…," she says, "that he has had…those chunks… of life."

As we sit in the courtyard I mention to Mom how two weeks ago today, before she fractured her pelvis, we celebrated her seventy-fifth birthday. I tell her that we had three celebrations. Ben and I and the kids took her out for dinner and gave her presents, then, on another day, Morgan and I brought a large ice cream cake to share with the residents and staff at Greenway.

"A lot of people really like you there, really care about you." When I tell her this, Mom smiles.

The third party was at the cottage with some of her old friends: Bill and Susan, more neighbors from along the lake, and two women who worked at the library and knew her for years. I wanted her friends to be able to celebrate her life, even if she recognized only a few of them, and to share her joy in their company. I had hoped to invite some of her oldest friends, but if she still had an address book with their phone numbers, I didn't find it when we moved her out of the cottage.

Today is the first time in over a year that I've gone to my support group. Until Mom's multiple hospital admissions this summer, things were going smoothly and I didn't feel a need to go. I recognize three women, all of whom have husbands with Alzheimer's disease. Arlene, a tall, elegant woman of seventy with bright-red lipstick and short, white hair, has a husband in the dementia ward of the nursing home where Mom is in rehab. He's farther along in his dementia than my mother, and he no longer speaks. Arlene visits him every day, but she tells us, "I know the man I visit is no longer the man I married." I assume that since Arlene is more experienced than I am she is absolutely right; I don't question her wisdom. I assume that my mother will also change into a different person. In fact, with her sudden struggle with words, I assume that the process has already begun. I equate language with self.

Slowing Down

After dinner on a Tuesday, I walk the three minutes it takes to get from our house to the large building in the center of our community that serves as a meeting space.

Thirty of us are here to listen to a presentation about how to support Rita, our one resident living with dementia. Rita has grown harder to understand, and over the past couple of years most of her neighbors have shied away from her, including me. Karen, a neighbor who leads the presentation, trains family caregivers and paid caregivers nation-wide in compassionate, person-directed care. Her father also had Alzheimer's disease. Beth, another neighbor who has helped Rita's children coordinate her care long-distance, joins her. A third neighbor and presenter, Adele, has spent a great deal of time with Rita as one of what they call her "care partners." I'm excited to learn all I can from these women and to perhaps share some of my own experiences.

"Instead of trying to change the behavior of someone living with dementia," Karen suggests, "focus on shifting your own expectations or shifting the environment. Look at what works now, their strengths rather than their limitations, and build on those."

Adele tells us, "If Rita says something that doesn't seem to make sense, try to find something that works with it. It's like a puzzle. You don't need to have a deep conversation to have a deep connection. Relax with it and don't worry about it." I think I can try this. I already try to work around my mother's odd choice of words.

"Affirm their reality," Karen says, "and creatively re-direct them if you need to steer the person away from insisting on something that isn't a good idea." Beth shares an example: If Rita wants a third serving of ice cream at a community meal because she doesn't remember how much she's already had, Beth doesn't try to reason with her. She tells her "We'll have ice cream at home." Rita says, "Okay," and within a few minutes forgets all about it.

Have I bent the truth with Mom? Not too often. Instead I try to explain reality as I see it, repeating myself over and over as she forgets what I've said. I resist lying to her to make things easier, not only because Mom is not yet that difficult to deal with, but also because I'm used to our honest relationship. Part of me worries that if I start bending the truth with Mom she will catch on and no longer trust me.

Karen explains that non-verbal communication is very important to people living with dementia. Talk to them at eye level, she says. I wonder if that's why Mom's physical therapist and nurse at Woodside crouched in front of her wheelchair to talk to her. I always lean over in front of her, never crouch or kneel, because of my arthritic knees.

Convey respect, she says. Use a low-pitched voice. Stay calm.

Karen talks about affirming the reality of people living with dementia. "If they tell you the sky is green, the sky is green. Don't try to change their perspective." Do I correct my mother when she says something that's clearly incorrect? I'm not sure. I could try harder to validate Mom's ideas and feelings.

"Paraphrase what she's said," Karen suggests. "Reflect back what you've heard to clarify your understanding of it."

Adele admits that paraphrasing can be challenging. "When I'm talking with Rita it's complicated. I have to think all the time."

Yes, I find it hard sometimes to follow Mom's train of thought. I have to concentrate, listen hard. I believe this is one of the main reasons why people avoid talking to those with dementia—the puzzle of their mixed-up language. It helps if you know the person well enough to guess what they are reaching for.

"One of the things I love about spending time with Rita," Adele says, "is that I can just be myself with her. Sometimes we worry that we have to act a certain way with people or they won't like us. With Rita you don't have to worry about what she thinks of you, because she's not thinking about you!" She laughs.

Karen agrees: "It's freeing."

"And when I'm with Rita," Adele adds, "she helps me slow down and notice so many wonderful things around us. She'll stop on our walks and study a leaf, or point to a bird in a tree. I call my hours with her 'the church of Rita.'"

The next day, a Friday, I visit Mom and carry with me what I learned the night before. I decide to see her after work not out of my usual worry and sense of duty, but simply to sit with her, to slow down and enjoy together whatever pleasure we can find.

Outside, as we sit in the courtyard together, I think of what Karen said last night about helping people with dementia feel useful; often people living with dementia are asked to do very little, to always receive care instead of giving care. I look into my mother's eyes and say, "Mom, I could really use a hug."

"Sure, sweetie!"

We hold onto each other a long time. I take her hands in mine.

"You have such strong hands," I say. "They're slender but strong." We lean toward each other, our faces a foot apart.

"So do you," she says as she smiles and caresses the freckles on my forearm. For a moment we look into each other's eyes.

"I love you," she says.

"I love you, too." Though I've forced myself to say it before, this time I mean it. I feel calm and relaxed, not wary and ready to flee.

Mom says, "The two of us…have come…a long way."

I smile and squeeze her hand. "Yes, we really *have* come a long way." Is she remembering what we used to be like together, how hard we've worked over the years to grow closer to each other? I want to cry when she says this. Does she really remember all those years, or is she just saying something polite that she might say to anyone she's known a long time?

"Let's keep going…in that…direction," she says. She's still smiling and looking deep into my eyes.

With this, I think she really does know what she's saying. And that's all I've ever wanted—"to keep going in that direction." I want us to grow closer, if only by annoying each other less and enjoying each other more.

"Yes, Mom, let's do that. I'd like that."

It's too late to work out any lingering resentments between us, as Mom can't remember the specifics of our conflicts. So I see no point in hanging on to them. The long-distance affection my mother and I used to share years ago through our letters and phone calls—the affection that, in person, cooled within minutes—now holds steady, for the most part, through our short visits together, warm and full.

A few moments later, though, Mom starts to squirm. "I'd like to… go in. I think I need to go…" and she points to her crotch.

I'm surprised that she can feel the need to go to the bathroom, as lately she hasn't seemed aware of her bodily needs, but I quickly stand up, circle her around and wheel her back inside to the bathroom in her room. Her new roommate, Edie, is not there, but I see a baby doll on the foot of Edie's bed. I point it out to Mom. I'm surprised, amused, a bit creeped out. The tiny doll, swaddled in a receiving blanket, looks like a newborn with its red, wrinkled face.

Standing ready to catch her if she falls, I watch Mom as she lifts herself out of the wheelchair, grabs the walker, and walks stiffly to the toilet. This is the first time I've helped with her Depends, the first time I've helped her do more in the bathroom than enter and leave. I worry that she'll feel embarrassed, but she seems quite comfortable.

When she finishes on the toilet, I grab a dry pair of Depends folded over the handrail next to us on the wall. They look way too big for Mom but I figure they're better than nothing. I remember reading online that if you are changing someone's Depends, do so from behind so they can't see what you are doing and you preserve their dignity. Mom doesn't seem at all concerned about her dignity. Nevertheless I stand a bit behind her as I lean down to tuck the front half of the Depends through her thighs ("Excuse me, let me just pull this through"), then reach around in front to pull them up to her navel. I fasten the sticky tabs, and Mom pulls up her pants.

"I don't like these much," she says, and I guess that she means because they're cumbersome, not because she objects to the idea of wearing protective undergarments. The more time I spend with her, the more I can intuit what she means. She zips up her pants, I point her toward the sink and the soap dispenser, and she slowly washes her hands. I remind myself to be patient. I crank down a paper towel and she meticulously dries her hands. "There's the waste basket," I say. "Yup, right there."

I watch closely as she shuffles with her walker to her wheelchair. I suggest that we go for a ride down the hall to the vending machine: I'll buy her a candy bar.

"Sure!"

I push her around a corner, down a hallway I doubt she has ever seen.

Mom twists in her seat to look back at me. "I'm nervous. I don't know...what's at the end...of where we are going...and where we came from."

With her words I inhale a sharp breath, and stop for a moment in the empty hallway. All I can do is touch her shoulder. "Don't worry, Mom. The staff lounge is just down here. We'll get some candy, and we'll come right back."

Old Friends

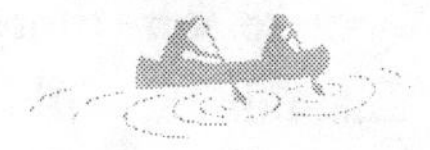

I spend Labor Day weekend at the cottage with Ben and the kids, and I don't feel guilty about not seeing Mom for a whole three days; in fact I don't think about her at all. I read the *Times*, watch the waves shift on the lake, and play cards with Ben and the kids and a friend of Andrew's. I barbecue chicken over a wood fire on the beach, and swim in the cool, shallow water. Physical labor relaxes me; I pull weeds out of the lake near the beach and trim the bushes in the yard. I notice, though, that I pack even my relaxation into a dense schedule.

The Tuesday after Labor Day I leave work early to attend Mom's first care plan meeting at the rehab center. In their meeting room, I find seven staff members clumped along the far edge of a large, oval table. They motion for me to sit at the other end.

Katherine, the social worker, says, "Your mom is doing pretty well, but she's been a bit combative the last couple of days." Immediately

I feel guilty about leaving Mom alone all weekend, and worry that she's mad at me, or scared. I wouldn't have thought Mom could sense the difference between a day in between visits and three days.

"She's refusing to cooperate sometimes, and won't talk to her aides," Katherine says. "The aide sat with her at dinner and your mom completely ignored her."

Abby counters by saying, "I haven't had any problems with Judy in physical therapy. I haven't seen that combativeness. If Judy's in pain, she'll lash out, but that's understandable. If she's uncooperative or nasty, ask her if she's in pain—if she's in pain right that minute." This sounds a lot like what I said to Abby over the phone after Mom's first PT evaluation.

Also, I think to myself, if Mom does not like you—if you seem unfriendly, if you are cool and detached, or condescending, she will pick up on that right away and ignore you or resist any requests or commands. Probably the aide's personality just rubbed her the wrong way, while the physical therapist and floor supervisor are more solicitous. The aide, scowling, sits beside me.

Peggy, the floor supervisor, suggests that they test Mom for a urinary tract infection, which can cause irritability.

Gloria, the nutritionist, says that Mom refused to eat one of her meals—just pushed it away. I remind them about her two bowel inversions.

I explain that every time I see Mom, I take a look at her stomach to see if it's enlarged. Peggy says that she will keep track of Mom's bowel movements. Gloria the nutritionist says that, overall, Mom's eating well, about fifty percent of her meals, and drinking a lot. She is eating her dessert first, but also half of the entrees.

Peggy says, "Our main concern, besides the recent combativeness, is the fact that your mom has figured out how to unhook herself from the clip alarm when she's in the wheelchair and is walking around when she shouldn't be, without assistance. We don't want her to fall. We want to keep her safe."

"Isn't there a pad alarm on her wheelchair?" I ask.

"No, she only has a pad alarm on her bed," Peggy says. "We're trying to order a smaller version for the wheelchair. Your mom has figured out how to take the whole alarm box off of the wheelchair. She carries it around in her hand."

I can't help cracking a small smile.

To protect Mom if she falls, Abby recommends a product called HipSaver®, a girdle-like undergarment with soft padded discs over the hipbones and tailbone. I never knew such a thing existed, and agree to let them order her some.

At this facility, staff members do not see family caregivers as peripheral; they are truly welcoming me as a member of my mother's care team. I'm beginning to realize, too, how very important it is to me that paid caregivers like these staff members see me as an informed and competent family caregiver—a good and thorough daughter who knows her mother better than anyone else. With this implied affirmation I sit a bit taller in my chair.

For the first time since she left the cottage, my mother's old neighbors, Susan and Bill, drive over to visit. Susan tells me on the phone afterward that they had a long visit and that Mom was excited, "maybe too excited." They "reached into her past" to find things to talk about, like her grandchildren.

When I see Mom next I ask her if she remembers seeing them.

"Oh, yes," she says. "They talked a lot. They were really excited." Mom flutters her fingers around her head to show how excited they were.

This makes me happy. I believe that she really does remember how she felt when they were here. Though she can't remember the content of their visit, she remembers the emotion.

Transitions

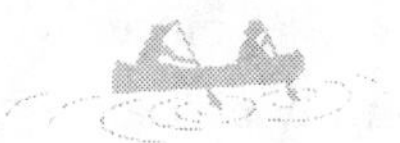

On a Thursday night, I join Arlene from my caregiver support group for a meeting of a different support group, this one for family members of Woodside residents. We will talk about the quality of the care our loved ones are receiving at Woodside, and any concerns we might have. Even though I have a cold, and Mom will be leaving rehab in a few weeks, I decide it's important to go to the meeting. If no one looks out for the care our family members receive in nursing homes and rehab centers, if no one checks up, we get what we deserve.

Several family members comment on how pleasant the home seems now that it has a new director. The first thing you notice, they say, is that it doesn't smell bad anymore. One man says, "If you don't notice anything, that means that everyone is doing their job."

The guest speaker for the meeting, the manager of the kitchen, says their motto is "residents and their families first," and tells us we can request any of eighteen diets—low fat, low salt, solid, soft, liquid, vegetarian, vegan, kosher. Arlene pipes up and says,

"I wonder why we allow our doctors to prescribe low-fat diets for our loved ones when food is one of the few pleasures left in their lives. I decided recently that my husband should be able to eat the foods he enjoys—pork chops, butter with his bread, ice cream." Good point, I think. But my mother is on a low-fat diet to help prevent more tiny strokes, and it doesn't occur to me for some time that more fat in her meals might help make them more enjoyable.

When the meeting ends I still feel like I have a low-grade fever, but I head downstairs and walk across the courtyard to the rehab center to see Mom for a quick minute. To my surprise, I find her sitting in her wheelchair right inside the double doors by the aides' station, facing the entrance, as if waiting for me or contemplating escape. She flings open her arms and we hug.

"Will you check my forehead, Mom?" I ask her. I feel like her little girl again. She rests her palm there for a moment. Her hand feels cool and smooth and soft.

"It's getting there!" she says, exactly as she used to.

Katherine, Woodside's social worker, asks me for permission to move my mother to the "secure" dementia ward in the nursing home section. "For the next couple of weeks that she's here," she says, "we want to keep your mom safe." Apparently Mom has been pushing her wheelchair through the rehab center's doors several times a day, sounding the alarm around her ankle and sending the staff running. I tell Katherine that's fine, Mom probably won't recognize that she's in a new room.

On my first visit to see her on the fourth-floor dementia ward, I step off the elevator into a large, white room, plain and antiseptic as a hospital, where two dozen residents sit at tables, silent. I note that the floor is clean and it doesn't smell. I see Mom by herself in a chair next to a table by the nurses' station. I'm pleased to see that she's out of the wheelchair and is again using a walker. When she spots me, she gives me a huge smile and raises her arms for a hug.

When she stands up to walk with me she pinches the sides of her pants at her hip.

"They're so...bunchy," she says.

I assume she's talking about the Depends, but maybe, I realize later, she's wearing the HipSavers that Abby recommended at the care plan meeting. Mom doesn't seem annoyed with them, just amused and maybe a little apologetic that her pants are puffy.

When we step into the elevator an alarm goes off. A middle-aged, female aide saunters over, shows me the combination to turn it off, and warns me that it will go off again when we get out on the first floor. I see the aide's slow movement as indifference; I haven't learned yet that moving slowly and calmly around a group of people living with dementia helps them feel safe and peaceful—and that moving slowly and deliberately helps the aides conserve their energy for a very long day. When the aide walks away and the doors close, Mom steps back toward the entrance of the elevator and the alarm goes off again. The aide returns to the elevator, stands facing Mom, puts her hands on Mom's shoulders, and pushes her backwards, away from the doors.

"You have to stand near the back, Judy, or the alarm will go off."

I can see that Mom is confused and a bit annoyed, but it all happens so fast that Mom doesn't have a chance to find the words to protest.

This is the first time I see my mother physically moved—pushed—from one spot to another. I would have explained to Mom that she needed to move back, and then I would have waited for her to move on her own. Or, if she hesitated, I would have taken her hand and asked her to step back with me. Obviously the aides don't have time to wait, but I still feel unsettled. I wouldn't blame her for getting "combative" at times if she's responding to this kind of treatment.

We walk outside to the courtyard, and Mom can move pretty well with the walker. It's a lovely mid-September day, just cool enough to need a light jacket, but sunny with a blue sky and soft white clouds. I'm not sure what to talk about. I realize for the first time that conversation usually relies on memory; no wonder I'm often at a loss for words when passing the time with Mom.

We're both content, though, to sit and enjoy the fresh air for a half hour, until she gets too cold. Upstairs I ask Mom to show me her new room, a single room with a bathroom and a pleasant view out the window of the same tree-lined street she could see from the rehab wing. The walls and floor look worn, old but not dirty. While the walls in the rehab center were painted homey colors like rose and peach, the walls here are a bland, eggshell white. This dementia ward, what some nursing homes call an Alzheimer's special care unit (SCU), apparently has no need to impress.

I don't want to leave my mother alone in such a threadbare place, surrounded by silent, mostly immobile patients in a more advanced stage of dementia, but she must stay and heal, and I must go.

Two days later, late in the afternoon on a Tuesday, I get a call from a woman at Woodside who identifies herself as the "Medicare coordinator." She tells me that the physical therapist reports that Mom has met all of her rehabilitation goals. Once a patient's goals are met, Medicare stops payment. Mom can stay at Woodside only through this Friday.

I'm taken by surprise, as only last week the staff thought Mom would be there a few more weeks. I will have three days to arrange Mom's transfer back to Greenway. What follows is a logistical debacle—missed doctors' signatures; delayed approvals from her old assisted living facility for her to move back; crises at my job; and Andrew's tenth birthday party. If Mom stays at the rehab center past Friday, there will be a high price to pay—$200, funds that Mom will need for her future care. Friday morning I squeeze two hours out of my day to move Mom back to Greenway.

I accept now that it's my job to look out for my mother, but I resist the weight of these sudden transitions. There are so many last minute demands from Greenway, that when I finally do get Mom back in her old room, I go into her bathroom and start to bawl. After a few minutes I force myself to stop or I'd be there all day and I wipe my face on some toilet tissue and walk back down to the TV room where Mom waits with Julia, a friend who also lives on her floor. I sit down next to my mother on the couch and Julia leaves. There is no one else in the room. I start to cry again. "Are you all right?" Mom asks.

"It's just been a hard day," I say. "I'm glad you're back and doing so well, but it's been hard."

I'm glad that she can listen. It feels good to cry next to her.

After a moment she says, "Just take care of you."

With these words, with her squeeze of my hand, I feel like I have my mother back again, and it's sweet. *But I can't take care of myself right now*, I think. *At least not today*.

As I leave I see Daphne, the case manager, who looks annoyed. I say, "I thought the only thing Mom needed to move back was the doctor's signature, as long as I arranged help."

"Well," Daphne says, following me to the door, "our staff hadn't decided yet whether she should move back. I was still checking. I tried to help you. I tried to be flexible. But maybe," she says, "I should just have said No."

"You don't know how many hoops I had to jump through today to get her back here!" I'm about to cry again.

"I know," she says softly.

"I give up!" I turn toward the parking lot, waving my arms at my side.

Inside my car I bawl again, this time not only overwhelmed, but ashamed. Still sitting in the parking lot, I call Maggie. My words come out in gasps. I tell her "Greenway doesn't seem too happy to have my mom back. I need to arrange help right away, at least first thing in the morning and at bedtime, maybe a check-in in the afternoon."

"No problem," Maggie says. "I have thirty-five girls working for me. I can have someone there right away."

I didn't realize she had a whole agency. Part of the reason I felt bad asking her for help at the last minute was because I thought she worked on her own.

"I'll come there myself, first thing in the morning, to see how your mom is doing. Don't worry. Everything will be all right."

The writing is, however, on the wall: Two days after I bring Mom back to Greenway, I get a call from Maggie. She has "serious concerns." Her aide found Mom at eight o'clock this morning "curled up in a ball" on her wet bed, her nightgown soaked up to the neck, no sheet or blanket over her. "Your mom's going to get a urinary tract infection," Maggie says. When she asked the RAs if they had Depends my mother could use they said they "didn't deal with that" (even though Daphne told me they could order them). So Maggie asked if she could borrow a few and then she'd buy some herself.

Last evening after dinner, she continues, no one could find Mom on the second floor. Maggie found her sitting alone in the auditorium on the first floor reading a magazine. "It's not safe," she tells me, "if no one has any idea where your mom is." She also did not have her walker. I know that Greenway is used to Mom being on the first floor, usually in the library. They don't panic unless she's invited into another resident's room and they can't find her.

Maggie tells me that all of this is "unfair to Judy." I never thought of it that way but she's right; Mom deserves better. Hesitating to offer her opinion unless asked, she does tell me that she prefers Maple Grove over Greenway because "all of the staff members are wonderful, caring and attentive. There is only one floor, and it's circular, so she wouldn't get lost. They're used to incontinence—ninety-five percent of the residents wear Depends. And they would check on her every hour at night." But Maggie doesn't like to see people "locked in" as they are in Maple Grove's dementia cottage, and suggests that I visit their other, unlocked, assisted living facility.

I trust Maggie's judgment about my mother's care more than anyone else's. She's worked for years in every elder care facility in our small city, and she's always been straight with me. Her aides seem reliable and kind. When Maggie offers to call the director at Maple Grove, a friend of hers, first thing in the morning to ask if they have a room available, I agree immediately. I haven't wanted to move Mom again, to make her get used to a new environment, but I'm so angry at Greenway right now. The image of my mother curled on her bed, wet and cold, turns me irrevocably against them.

It's time to move on. Carefully, yes, but quickly.

Part IV

MEMORY CARE

A Toss of the Dice

The main assisted living building at Maple Grove has no room available, but their dementia cottage, called Elm Haven, has one room free. I had preferred the main assisted living building, but I am desperate, now, to move my mother.

On Thursday I meet with Crystal, Elm Haven's sales director, for a tour in the late afternoon. When I arrive I watch through the window in the locked front door as she punches a code into a pad on the wall to let me in. My immediate impression of the cottage is that it's much more inviting than I'd imagined two years ago when I declined a tour, with its cozy living room, wall-to-wall rose carpeting, a gas fireplace with a fluffy white cat lounging on the hearth, and lots of natural light and plants. Six or seven women sit beside the fire, one reading a newspaper while the others listen to classical piano on a CD player. Everyone looks peaceful. Down a hall there's a room with a pool table for visiting family members, a small library, and a room for the hairdresser. The dining room, a tenth the size of the cavernous dining room at Greenway, is split into three small spaces. Two RAs, women in their thirties and forties, zigzag through the tables setting up for dinner.

Over the next few months I will learn that Elm Haven's staffing and design are typical of "memory care" assisted living facilities for people who have dementia but do not yet need a nursing home. While Elm Haven has half the number of residents as Greenway's conventional assisted living home, thirty compared to sixty, Elm Haven has five RAs on each shift compared to Greenway's two. "Memory care" staff provide much more hands-on care and individual attention. Nurses are also available twenty-four hours a day, compared to just the day shift nurse at Greenway. All staff members receive training, similar to what we learned in our intentional community's discussion of dementia, on how to interact with the residents to avoid triggering frustration or aggression.

I ask Crystal if residents ever receive medication to make them more compliant. "We try to avoid that at all costs," she says. "Usually we find that we can avoid any agitation in the first place with the right approach."

While activities at Greenway seem geared mainly toward the facility's independent residents, Elm Haven residents enjoy a full-time, bubbly and dedicated woman named Vicki who plans a daily roster of games, exercise classes, and other entertainment. Much of the activity, such as trivia quizzes and sing-a-longs, stimulates long-term memory.

The building lies on one floor, and hallways flow in a circle so residents can walk for as long as they want without getting lost. Beyond the generous windows there are two outdoor patios in the middle of the circle; in good weather the doors to the patios are always unlocked, with residents free to roam through the gardens or sit in the shade of an umbrella. Garden beds raised waist-high allow the residents to help the activities director plant tomatoes and basil. A screened-in porch holds wicker rocking chairs, and a canary and a parrot perched in cages.

Crystal shows me the available room on the other side of the dining room in a hallway called "Neighborhood C." It happens to be one of their largest single rooms, the most expensive. The room is very nice—freshly painted in ivory, with light blue-gray carpeting, a twin bed, side table, bureau, and a bathroom. The large windows look out over the parking lot, but in the distance I can see the lake. As we leave the room, Crystal points out a nook in the wall in the hallway next to the door, a cube-shaped space covered with Plexiglas called a "memory box," another common feature in memory care, where family members can put photos and memorabilia; for residents who can't read their names on the doors anymore, these displays serve as a way for them to recognize their rooms. Down the hall, there's another small living room, this one with fewer windows and a bit dark, with a couch and wingback chairs, a TV, and another canary.

I'm sure family members are supposed to find the design appealing, but I reserve judgment. I don't want to be sucked into thinking it's a wonderful place based on how it looks, when what will be most important is the quality of my mother's care and her daily enjoyment of life.

Crystal and I sit in one of the small dining rooms to talk. I've brought a list of all of Mom's major issues and review them with her. What I'm watching for is Crystal's skill at communicating—whether she's vague or frank.

"At what point, exactly," I ask, "would my mother have to move out?"

"Residents must be able to feed themselves, and be able to walk for at least a few steps, for example from the bed to a wheelchair."

That's the kind of answer I'm looking for. No gray areas.

She tells me that Elm Haven is applying for an "enriched" assisted living license from the state so residents would not have to leave when they could no longer do these two things. I assume these licenses take a while, so I don't hold my breath that Mom would benefit. (I will find out, five years later, that the state has still not ruled on Elm Haven's application—a tragedy for all of the residents who could have afforded to stay at Elm Haven but were forced into a nursing home in order to receive a little extra help.)

Crystal tells me that an RA would bring Mom's medication to her, in her room or wherever she is.

Great! I think. No more waiting in line.

When I mention Mom's bed railing she tells me Elm Haven is not allowed to use one because they're not a nursing home. I wonder why Greenway allowed it. (Maybe they didn't, and that's why it ended up in the closet.) She tells me they would push one edge of the bed against the wall, and tuck a long body pillow under the blanket along the other edge to create a bump to prevent her from rolling out. She says Elm Haven has a complex "fall management" system. In my eagerness to cover all my questions I forget to ask her to explain what she means.

Can they put an alarm pad on Mom's bed to alert the staff when she gets out of bed by herself? As they are not a nursing home, she says, they're not allowed to use them. They could put a soft pad on the floor to cushion her if she falls, she says, but the downside is that it's an unstable surface and might make it more likely that Mom would fall once she's standing. I agree to forgo the floor pad.

She tells me they can take Mom to her doctors' appointments if needed, for an extra charge. I tell her I will usually do that as I can answer all of the doctors' questions.

A podiatrist comes in every sixty days, she continues. I find this inordinately exciting, as it means I'll no longer have to take Mom out to get her toenails cut.

I tell her I'm interested in the one available room, but ask that Mom be put on a waiting list for a small private room or a shared room (which are quite large), to save her about $700 a month. We calculate that her monthly bill, including extra services such as supervision with toileting, and extra cleaning because of the incontinence, will come to $4,172. In comparison, her room at Greenway, the smallest they had available, came to $2,400 a month, but did not include the extra help she has needed from private aides, which, at $18 an hour for a few hours a week, added another $2,000 a month.

Crystal tells me that Elm Haven will also require a $4,000 one-time "community fee" to help pay for improvements to the common space such as new furniture and carpeting. I narrow my eyes and nod. That's a lot of money, but I like the fact that everything looks new and spotless.

In order to hold the room I will need to drop off all of her paperwork (social and medical history), plus a check for $8,172.10, first thing the next morning.

Crystal tells me they will visit Mom at Greenway and do an assessment. If we decide to go ahead, Ben and I can move Mom the following Tuesday.

I tell Crystal I'll let her know my decision first thing in the morning. Even with Maggie's recommendation, the onus is on me, no one else. I could get it right, or wrong.

Friday morning I throw the dice, cash out more of Mom's dwindling mutual funds, and deliver the check.

Moving Day

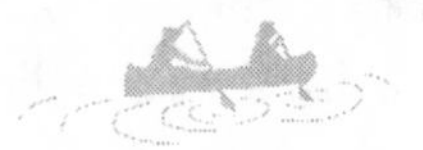

Ben has taken the day off from work to help me, and while I finished various errands, he's already emptied Mom's desk and drawers into boxes and packed up her clothes.

When Mom wakes up from a nap in front of the TV, I stop and sit with her and explain our plan. One of Mom's private aides sits beside her.

"We're going to have a bit of an adventure today," I say. "We're moving you to a really nice place where you'll get more help."

"I need help?" she says.

"Yes, you do, Mom." I don't know how to sugarcoat it. "You're incontinent—and that's okay—but you need help all the time now to make sure that you're clean and dry."

"Oh."

"The new place is only three minutes away from us! It's really, really nice, just like here, but we won't—you won't—have to pay extra for the help you need."

"I won't have to pay...?" She seems startled at the thought that any of this is costing her money.

"Yes, you won't have to pay extra. The new place will be just as nice but less expensive."

Mom nods slightly, her eyes wide.

A few residents stroll over to say good-bye. One woman has tears in her eyes and says, "Your mom is a great lady."

Another stops me as I escort my mother to the door. "I wanted to say good-bye, Judy." She clasps Mom's hand and Mom smiles at her.

The woman twists toward me and says, "I hate it when people move out and nobody tells us. And the staff can never give us a forwarding address. We sit together at meals and get to know each other, then all of a sudden your friend is gone! It's just not right."

"I know, I agree," I whisper to her. "But I didn't want to make it harder for my mother by walking around with her saying good-bye over and over. I'd have to keep explaining, and she might start to feel confused or anxious. You understand, right?"

I feel defensive again. There are so many choices, so many needs of other people to consider. In this case, by making the move easier for Mom by not saying a dozen goodbyes, I'm making it easier for myself as well, placing my needs in front. I'm pacing myself for another long day.

Settling In

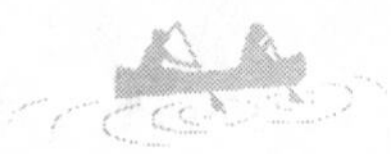

Oh, please let Elm Haven be the haven we need. I have been so stressed; I have been overeating—bits of Ben's birthday cake, anything I could get my hands on. If I can't get Mom safe and settled, I could end up weighing three hundred pounds.

As I meet with the staff, my thought is as intense as a prayer: *Let me like you.*

The head nurse at Elm Haven, Michelle, is a tanned, fit, and upbeat redhead in her forties who looks like an athlete. When we arrive, she trots out to the living room in her khakis and sneakers to greet us, and squats down in front of Mom's chair. She looks deep into Mom's eyes, and gives her the signature smile that we learn will always light up a room.

"Welcome, Judy!" she says. "I think you're really going to like it here!"

Though I'm still on hyper alert, ready to catch mistruths and false promises, her enthusiasm reassures me, at least at this moment, that all will be well.

In her new room, Mom sits in a cushioned rocking chair by the window to rest and watch us work. Ben unloads the van while Candy and I unpack her things. I notice for the first time that there is no tub or shower in her bathroom, only the toilet and sink. I ask the maintenance man where the shower is and he points down the hall. Hmmm, I think, just like a dormitory. I feel sad for a moment that Mom won't need the lovely cloth shower curtain I gave her to use at Greenway.

Various staff members come in to chat with Mom. The housekeeper introduces herself, and Michelle comes back several times to check that Mom has everything she needs. As we unpack, an elderly man shuffles in Mom's open door and stands staring at Mom. He's pale but has chiseled features and a full head of salt-and-pepper hair. I say hello and tell him that Mom—"her name is Judy"—is new, she's moving in today. Though his face lies slack, his eyes betray a hint of amusement and curiosity. He stares another moment, silent, then turns and shuffles out. I look over at Mom: She's wide-eyed and squirming.

"I guess people kind of wander around," I say. "Maybe he wanted to say hello."

Mom shakes her head and purses her lips. "I don't like that," she says.

Mom pushes herself up from the chair and walks to the bed, lies down on top of the quilt, pulls off one sneaker, and closes her eyes. I pull off the other sneaker, but when Mom is almost asleep, the director, Diane, knocks and comes in. She's a tall, middle-aged woman with dark-rimmed glasses and short, blonde hair.

"Is that you?" she asks my mom about a blown-up, framed photo we've hung on the wall over Mom's bed of me at eighteen, the one where Mom hired a professional photographer. It was a cool day in March and I'm up in a tree, standing on the thick fork of its trunk, my arm draped on a branch; my hair is brown and short, layered in a Dorothy Hamill cut; my smile and the knowing look in my hazel eyes both impish and mature beyond my years.

"Yes, that's me," Mom says.

"No, it's me," I say. I can't keep myself from correcting her on this one; I am not my mother and she is not me. And has she forgotten what I looked like?

Diane asks about another photo on the wall, the blown-up, framed photo of Mom canoeing around her lake. "Did you live on Silver Lake?" she asks, referring to the history I provided on Mom's intake papers.

"No, never," Mom says with conviction.

"You lived in the cottage on Silver Lake for twenty-five years," I interject. To Diane, I say, "Mom's getting tired." Doesn't the staff realize, I wonder, how exhausting this kind of long day is for someone with dementia?

At 5:30 it's time for dinner in her new home, so with her walker, Mom and I make our way the few feet to the dining room while Candy eats her bagged meal in Mom's room. Mom and I will have the smallest, "family" dining room all to ourselves, with its centerpiece of plastic leaves and pumpkins. Dinner disappoints us, though, and Mom eats little except for dessert. The director stops to chat.

"You're probably just tired, Judy. Maybe tomorrow you'll wake up with more of an appetite." I like that the director checked on us. I feel confident that tomorrow they'll make sure she eats. She'll be fine. *Won't she?*

As I leave I feel the same as the day I left Mom at Greenway after her stint at the rehab center: sad and empty, but light-headed with relief.

A week after Mom moves in, Maggie calls me again. Whenever she calls, my anxiety rises in anticipation of a problem. The first thing she tells me, though, is good news. The day before, Candy, the aide, drove Mom to the Friends of the Library book sale, to the park, and out to lunch. Mom "had a great time." But when Candy had arrived at eight a.m., Maggie says, she found Mom in bed asleep with her clothes on, as if she hadn't been dressed for bed the night before, and wearing a soaking wet Depends.

The Elm Haven RAs keep a log of their notes in the room, and the previous night's log said that Mom has been doing some kicking and hitting. Maybe that's why she wasn't changed. Maggie suggests that I "keep on them about the hygiene stuff." She also offers to have her aide give Mom a shower on the days she's there, as Elm Haven charges extra for showers beyond two days a week.

Diane, the director, tells me that Mom has been agitated, or "restless," as she prefers to call it, as it's a new place and she doesn't know anyone, and the staff are used to that. If she was kicking and hitting Sunday night, she says, they would have left her alone and let her sleep in her clothes. Diane will check the records for that night, but we are more concerned about the wet Depends. "It might break down her skin," I say, and she agrees.

I tell Diane that Michelle, the nurse, has called me already with a few concerns and that I appreciate the clear communication. I tell her they can call me at any time. Diane says that likewise if I have any concerns I can call them at any time, day or night. This is a welcome change from Greenway.

I also tell Diane that Maggie's outside aides will be tapering off next weekend, that after this initial period of adjustment they will be coming only once a week, for about six hours, to take Mom out.

I need to order Mom more HipSavers online. Also, a prosthesis for her mastectomy. The prosthesis seemed to get lost when she went to the hospital in the summer when I was out of town on vacation. When she first lost it, she would pat her chest and laugh as if to say that something was missing. Though she doesn't seem to notice its absence now, I still want to make sure that my mother has everything she would have ordered for herself a few years ago—the same kind and color of Keds, the same high-necked, ruffled nightgowns she liked because they hid her mastectomy, those ubiquitous, ivory trouser socks. I don't care if my mother's shirts lie concave on one side (both sides are pretty flat now, anyway), but I would feel guilty if I didn't provide, with her checkbook, the kinds of personal products and clothing she used to care about very much.

I am soon increasingly impressed with Elm Haven. They have ordered a different style of Depends—the kind in one piece, like underwear, without the side tabs that made it so easy for Mom to rip them off. No more waking up wet in bed. Problem solved.

Living Grief

In late October, two and a half years since she moved in with us, I bring Mom along with me and Ben and the kids for an afternoon at the lake. I imagine that she will light up at the sight of the cottage, but as she sits outside with me in the front yard in the shade of an umbrella, and watches the waves, her expression is flat, muted, as if the yard is just a place like any other.

At first, I feel deflated, but within moments I realize something: It's time for me to stop trying to bring my mother pleasure through what's left of her memory. If she no longer recognizes the deep blue swell of her lake, if these pieces of her life no longer move her, then truly there's nothing but the present moment—and other people.

I decide to take her out for a rowboat ride. We had asked a boat builder in Maryland to make the forest-green rowboat, in the same color and style as I remember my grandfather's old boat. I wonder if feeling the rowboat rock softly on the water will help my mother experience the joy in the lake she used to feel in her canoe, or when she watched the waves from her desk.

Ben helps me support Mom under her arms as she steps in. Mom sits in the middle of the wide seat along the back of the boat, Andrew squeezes into the bow, and from the middle seat I row the three of us a hundred feet out into the lake. I keep my eyes on hers. She grips the edge of the seat, her back ramrod straight, her eyes wide but not scared. We bounce gently on the waves and Mom releases her hands from the seat to stretch her arms and clasp the sides of the boat. She smiles. When I tell her that she can lean against the high back wall of the boat, she scoots her bottom toward the wall and relaxes.

Back on shore, there's a problem. We find that Ben has gone off to the store; Andrew and I have to pull up the heavy boat and get Grammy out on our own. I call Morgan out of the house for her help. We hold Grammy's hands and coach her to walk up the length of the boat from the back, which is still in the water, to the bow so we can help her step out onto the beach. She stands on the seat in the bow, too high to step down. I ask Andrew and Morgan to find a stool in the boathouse and they bicker about who should go. Andrew finds my garden stool, which has wheels, and I wedge it between my feet beside the boat and try to persuade Mom to step down on it.

"Don't make me cry," she says.

My heart flares for a moment with guilt, but she trusts me and her fear passes quickly. She holds my hands firmly as I ask Andrew to carry over one of the lawn chairs. Mom hesitates, then lifts one leg over the rail of the boat and steps onto the chair, brings her other leg over, pauses, then steps down to the garden stool and then onto the shale, where she tucks her slender shoulders into my arms. Such a production! I can't believe I asked my mother, who just recovered from a pelvic fracture, to clamber in and out of a boat.

But I'm glad I did. In the boat Mom seemed to absorb it all—my attention as I held her eye and smiled at her, the breeze, the blue-green waves, the gentle push of the oars, the firmness of the boat's floor under her Keds. When we passed our neighbors on their dock Mom had let go of the side of the boat to wave with a big smile.

Without memory, I think to myself, what's left? Not destinations like going to the cottage—not the pleasure of their anticipation and repetition—but moments like these, of sense and touch, rhythm and movement, patience and reassurance.

The rest of our hours together on this visit feel more strained. As Mom sits in the living room she looks bored, flips through a few books and reads out loud to me the same titles over and over. I offer her grapes and juice then worry that she'll knock her glass off the arm of the chair where she balances it so I carry the juice back and forth to her from the kitchen table. Andrew and Morgan play board games on the living room rug with frequent exclamations and rough-housing, and I worry that Mom will get up and walk around when I'm not looking and trip on something or weave and fall down; we brought her walker but she forgets to use it. I scan the floor for the kids' sneakers and other tripping hazards. I worry that she will try to go outside for a walk and fall down the concrete stairs. Ben and I serve lunch but she picks at her food.

I ask her if she has to go to the bathroom and she says yes and points to the brass carrier in front of the fireplace used to haul wood. "I'll just go in that," she says.

I do a double take, mildly disgusted. "No, Mom, I'll help you use the toilet."

"Are you sure...I can't...just go in that?"

"No, I'm sure. You need a toilet."

Later, as we sit in the living room, I ask Mom, "Do you like being here, Mom, at the cottage?"

"Yes…if those who are here…are not…in a tangle." Her eyes flash annoyance, her tone so much like years ago.

Maybe the kids' bugging each other upsets her, but I can't tell. I'm not sure what she wants. Is it not enough that we invited her to join us today? I decide not to respond, though, to let it go. I leaf through a magazine left by a renter and find an article by Lauren Kessler, journalist and author of the book *Dancing with Rose: Finding Life in the Land of Alzheimer's*, about the three months she spent working as an RA in a memory care facility similar to Elm Haven. She writes that people with Alzheimer's disease often become hypersensitive to the emotions of others. Certainly my mother seems hypersensitive, I think. If I am not bouncing with cheeriness at every moment, if I relax my body, the muscles in my face, if I dull my eyes and drift off into my own thoughts, as I try to do now, Mom seems to take it as rejection.

Mom stands up and heads for her coat. "I'm ready to go."

"We'll leave soon," I lie. "Please sit down." I no longer mind bending the truth to keep my mother calm.

What I haven't learned yet is to keep our visits extremely short—just an hour or two. An entire afternoon is really too much for both of us.

Later in the evening, at home in the kitchen, I thank Andrew for his help with the boat ride, and give him a hug. An insightful young man of few words, he says, "I can see why Grammy is such a handful."

If, in the wee recesses of my mind, I was still entertaining the idea of saving Mom's money by taking care of her myself at our house again, this afternoon at the cottage convinced me that I don't have the stamina. The experience finally, completely, vanquished the guilt.

For my birthday at the end of October, Ben brings home a dozen red roses and a box of chocolates, and Morgan gives me a handmade card, plus two novels and a heart-shaped necklace she found in our community's re-use room (the "free pile") that she thought I would like. I'm sick with a cough and low-grade fever and don't want to go out anywhere. Since I became a caregiver, I've had bronchitis every few months. I have to inhale a steroid twice a day to prevent more frequent infections. As the women in my caregiver support group warned me early on, caregivers often get sick. But I won't make the connection between the stress and my illness, or begin to feel better, for several years.

As the late afternoon sun pierces the gaps between the blinds, I sit at the kitchen table and call my mother.

The RA who answers the office phone tells me that Mom is "watching some entertainment. Are you sure you want to interrupt her?" Yes, I'm sure.

Mom picks up on an extension. I say hello.

"Hi, sweetheart!" she exclaims.

"I just wanted to say hi because today's my birthday."

"It is? I'm so sorry, I forgot."

"That's okay. I just wanted my mommy to wish me a happy birthday."

"Happy birthday!" she says with a laugh.

I tell her I would have come over to see her but I didn't want to get her sick. "When I feel better I'll come over and we'll go out to celebrate my birthday."

"When will that be?"

"Maybe I'll feel better in a few days," I say, then add, "I sure wish I could get a big birthday hug!"

"I would give you...*five hundred* hugs!" she says.

"I know, Mom." I'm smiling inside, but don't know what else to say. "Can you believe I'm forty-three today?"

"Forty-three?" she says, incredulous.

"Yeah. When did that happen?"

"I don't know!" She laughs. After a pause she says, "I bet you have a lot going on."

"Not really. I'm not doing much today because I'm sick. In a couple days I'll come see you."

"I'd like that. I'd like that...real big!" She laughs again.

I don't know what else to talk about so I say, "It sounds like your tongue is still dry." Mom's incontinence medication, which she started a week ago, has the side effect of dry mouth. Her lips and tongue are parched, shriveled. When she's not sipping a drink, she talks with a lisp.

"It is. It weally is."

"Maybe it will wear off," I say. "We'll check with Dr. Claiborne."

"That would be great, because my mouth is weally dry."

"I'll let you go now, Mom. I'll see you soon. I love you."

"I love you, too, honey. See you soon."

It may sound childish, but when I hang up I feel as if I have lost my mother—in a new, irrevocable way. Sometimes I feel that she's still there, and sometimes she's a new, more loving and forgiving mother, but this time, in this moment, I feel as if I have lost, not gained; I've lost the mother who would always remember to call and sing me "Happy Birthday," the one who would buy me books she knew I'd enjoy, the one who made me angel food cake with fluffy pink marshmallow frosting, the one who sent me home-made cards on my birthday and Valentine's Day with red hearts and X's and O's. On days such as today I need her, my mother who remembers me and shows me she loves me through particular things, certain traditions. I'm not ready to give her up. I sit at the table and cry.

In the Moment

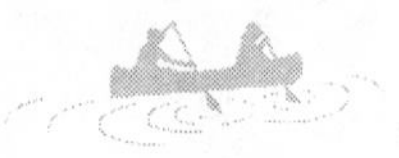

The next Sunday, when I feel better, I explain to Ben and the kids that I'm going to take Mom out for my birthday, just the two of us, "because it's easier that way and no one is unhappy." I feel a bit guilty not including them, but know that the kids would grow restless with how long it takes Mom to do everything, and Ben would be bored. And I know that I will enjoy lunch more if I allow myself to focus my attention on her.

When I called Elm Haven yesterday to tell them that I would be coming today to take my mother out, Crystal, the staff member who gave me the tour, answered the phone, and told me, "Your mom is such a sweetheart—always so pleasant." She had a really nice chat with Mom the day before, and Mom told her, "Let's do this again some time—real soon." Crystal suggested to Mom that they "make a date" for the following day; she's planning on sitting down with Mom for a chat, as planned, even though Mom would not recall talking about it, "because I would remember," she said. Though I'm glad that Mom is getting this kind of attention, I remain cautious; Crystal's interest in my mother feels fake. Maybe this feeling comes from the fact that Crystal is the facility's sales director.

I walk down the hallway past my mother's room to the dark TV room at the end of her wing. She's sitting on the couch, staring down at the carpet with a concerned look on her face, ignoring the TV. Her hair is completely flat, lying straight down from a part in the middle, greasy-looking. I feel annoyed that they didn't wash her hair when they gave her a shower this morning, but then I realize that it's not dirty, it's just wet.

It's early November, cold, and I wonder why the RAs think it's all right to leave her hair wet when she's about to go out. I ask Mom if she'd like me to blow-dry her hair. I walk her down to her room and ask her to sit. I plug in the blow dryer she's owned for years, an ancient, bulky model, very loud.

"Mom, when I was little you used to take me with you when you got your hair cut. You used to tell me that your hair was so thick it always surprised the hairdresser how long it would take them to blow it dry."

"Sure!" She laughs—tickled, I think, that I remember.

Tentatively, with my fingers, I lift the layers of her hair to dry underneath, brushing my fingertips against her scalp. I've never touched my mother like this. I used to brush my great-grandmother's hair, but never my mother's. Her head feels tiny to me, fragile like blown-out eggshell. As I touch her, I hold my breath.

At the restaurant, I show Mom how to use her fork to spear the rings of calamari. She doesn't seem to know which utensil to use unless it's the only one in front of her. She also doesn't seem to know what to do with her napkin; I show her how to put it on her lap. A few months ago she would have had no problem with these things.

Mom barely eats anything, and I wonder if she eats this little at Elm Haven, whether an RA sits at her table and encourages her and her tablemates to eat, or if she is left alone to waste away. I am amazed she is not thinner around the face and arms. I understand why family members, usually a spouse or partner, visit their loved ones in nursing homes and assisted living places at meal time to encourage their loved ones to eat. I consider doing that for Mom, but she seems to be strong so I decide that for now it's unnecessary and I don't have the time.

As we wait for dessert, Mom reaches across the table to hold my hand. She smiles.

Years ago, Mom rarely touched me without annoying me. If she wanted to tell me something and I wasn't quite paying attention she'd look me in the eye and push three fingers into my forearm. I don't think she meant anything by it, but the pressure felt a bit too intense and controlling, and it made me recoil. Now when she reaches for me it's just to hold my hand, touch my cheek, or stroke my freckles.

"I like this," she says. I think she means the two of us, together.

"I do, too, Mom." I love these brief moments when there's nothing to do or explain, when we can just sit together.

I sit back and let her eat most of the cake, ice cream, and whipped cream, a serving for two. At least I'll get some calories into her. The waitress says to my mother, "You have a wonderful daughter." To me she says, "You are so patient."

Sure, I think, I can be patient for a few hours every week or so. I couldn't do this every day. I feel my chest grow warm. I'm not what this waitress thinks I am. I'm a fraud. A *real* caregiving daughter would take her mom out more than once every week or two. She'd be hands-on nearly every day. No—a *real* caregiving daughter would take care of her mother every day, in her own home. My saintly patience is fake.

Later, of course, I come to my senses. I reject whatever expectations strangers—or even the staff at Elm Haven—might have about what I should do or be as a daughter. I know that I am a true caregiver, whether I live five minutes away from my mother or five hours; whether I see her every day or once a year; whether I help her shower and cut her meat or let someone else. I accept that what I choose to do is enough. It's more than enough.

When I pay the bill and ask Mom to stand up, she clutches her cloth napkin.

"Should I bring this?" she asks. Every time we leave a place—a restaurant, my house, my van—Mom looks around to see what she brought with her, what belongs to her, picking up things at random as if she owns them, reluctant to put them down.

I decide to answer her using language I learned in a parenting class when Andrew was three and Morgan still a baby. Instead of saying, "You need to pick up your toys" or "Please shut the door," you use less bossy, less confrontational language: "The toys need to be picked up" or "The door needs to be closed."

"The napkin needs to stay here," I say. "The waitress will take care of it."

It works. Mom nods, and drops the napkin.

Back at Elm Haven, we take a walk.

"Isn't it nice to have such a lovely old barn right next to you?" I ask Mom.

"Oh, yes," she says, but she's looking the other way. We continue around another corner of the building where a vast section of a dairy farm lies planted in clover, an expanse of emerald unblemished by houses or pavement.

"Isn't this a beautiful field to have right next to you?" I ask, sounding to myself like a bit of a simpleton, but Mom agrees again. I can tell, though, that she's not really looking, not really appreciating it. Maybe she's getting tired. Why do this, then? Because I'm still trying to include in my mother's life things she used to love. As with the ride in the rowboat I want Mom to feel the breeze, and see all the colors around her. I'm disappointed in her reaction, but comforted that her new home lies surrounded by beauty.

As we continue I point out a tall lattice fence that encloses one of the two inner courtyards. To prevent residents from wandering outside, the gate on the fence is padlocked.

Mom looks up at a wisteria vine running along the top of the fence, its dried blossoms like clusters of grapes.

"I like that," she says.

I knew you would, I think to myself, and smile.

In her room Mom takes a look around as if she's never been here before. "This is nice!" I steer her to the toilet and gently pull down her layers. Usually when I visit now I leave it to the RAs to help her in the bathroom. I feel guilty about this, lazy, as if my discomfort—and boredom—with such tasks are a moral failure. I know that family members who take care of their loved ones at home face this task routinely with skill and patience, but I remind myself that my mother would never have wanted me to spend our visits wiping her bottom.

I notice today some evidence that she might be developing bowel incontinence, but I immediately push the thought out of my mind. It's too sad. I help her change so she won't get a urinary tract infection.

I leave Mom sitting in the main living room with a copy of the Sunday *Times* magazine. I push the door open and look back to catch her eye and wave good-bye. She waves back and sends a big smile across the room. As I wave to her, I sense a dozen pairs of eyes watching us; this room full of strangers seems to intrude on what should be our private moment of affection.

Home after only four hours away, I'm drained. For my sake our time together could have been shorter, but I knew I had not seen her for two weeks, and a shorter visit would have felt to me as if I were cheating her, taking advantage of her poor memory, pulling a fast one.

Today I noticed that Mom never used my name. She introduced me to another resident at Elm Haven as "my daughter," and when I told the woman my name was Martha, Mom perked up and said "Yes, this is Martha," as if she had forgotten. Usually she introduces me as "my daughter, Martha"—but not today. I wonder if she's reached the point where she will remember our relationship but not my name.

I don't realize yet that each day will be different, and if she doesn't use my name it might be temporary.

Shock and Awe

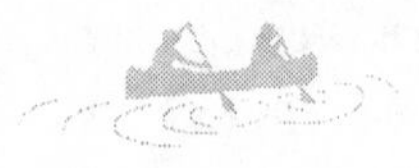

Today is Mom's first care plan meeting at Elm Haven, her thirty-day review, and I'm not sure what to expect. While I wait in the early afternoon for my appointment to begin, I find Mom in the main dining room, standing alone and looking disheveled and blurry-eyed.

"Oh, honey, what are you doing here?" she exclaims, and reaches for a hug. I say that I'm here to see the nurse. I don't explain that I'm also seeing the director and that it's a meeting about her.

An RA named Carrie, a blonde woman in her thirties who is always friendly and helpful, emerges from the locked kitchen carrying a plate of food, which she sticks in the microwave. She explains to me that Mom just woke up.

"She's been getting up later and later the last few days," she says, "fighting with us when we try to wake her up. We had a meeting about it this morning. They told us"—meaning the director and the nurse, I assume—"that if your mom's irritable, to let her sleep until she's ready to get up."

Immediately I feel stressed. If Mom is sleeping in until two o'clock in the afternoon, I think to myself, she's missing two meals and most of the day's activities.

The RA adds, "I'm not happy that they're letting her sleep all day, and I told them so."

Thanks for letting me know, I say. I admire her willingness to talk to me frankly and to tell her superiors what she thinks. On the legal pad I'm carrying, I add "sleeping in" to the list of issues I want to talk about at the meeting.

I sit with Mom at her table while she picks at her lunch. She starts to gag on a piece of beef. Adrenaline shoots through me, and I'm ready to do the Heimlich maneuver, but she's okay. We're alone in the dining room. If she eats by herself at odd hours, I think, what happens if she chokes for real and no one is around? Difficulty swallowing can be a symptom of advancing Alzheimer's disease.

Diane, the director, comes to get me for our meeting, and with a kiss I tell Mom that I will be back to see her in a few minutes. In the library I sit in one of the wingback chairs by the closed French doors, across the room from Diane and Michelle, the head nurse. I like Michelle a great deal—she's conscientious and thorough. I haven't had much experience with Diane, but she's friendly enough.

Diane asks me, "So how do you think it's been going?"

"Very well in general," I say. I bring up the over-sleeping. Yes, they say, your mom has been sleeping late the last few days, but it hasn't been going on long. She refuses to get up by ten o'clock or eleven, when she was generally getting up, and she's staying up until about two or three in the morning. Michelle says that Mom is also not sleeping well when she is in bed; she gets up, turns on the lights, and goes back to bed on top of the covers, sideways.

I ask them, "Aren't sleep disturbances normal for later phases of dementia?" I ask them what they do for other residents. Apparently if the family prefers it, the resident may need to be given a sleeping pill.

I don't mind the idea of a sleeping pill at all, but when they say it would be a narcotic I say, "If Mom were in her right mind she would never want to take a narcotic because she's a recovering alcoholic." At least I think she would not want to take it; I'm not sure. She once told me that her local 12-step group twenty years ago was "too strict" about avoiding medication. The taboo against medication made her put off seeking chemical help for her depression and anxiety.

Diane tells me, "We will respect your mother's wishes. If she would not have wanted a narcotic before the dementia, we will not give it to her."

"Could you give us a bit of history of your mom's sleeping patterns?" Michelle asks me. "Has she always been a restless sleeper? Has she always tended to stay up late and sleep in?" She leans forward and looks in my eyes. I tell them that as far as I know Mom slept well at Greenway but rarely got up before ten a.m. I warn them that if left to her own devices she will probably stay on the schedule she kept when she lived alone at the cottage three years ago, staying up half the night and sleeping until noon or later. I tell them I would prefer—I would just feel better—if Mom stayed on a more normal schedule. "I'd like to know she's part of the regular daytime world," I say.

We agree to monitor Mom's sleeping patterns for a few more weeks before deciding whether or not to use a sleeping aid. They could also start, Michelle says, with just a Tylenol to help her sleep. I ask her to try that.

I tell them I'm concerned that if Mom misses breakfast and lunch she won't get enough to eat. And if she's sleeping through many of the daytime activities, I say, "There is no point in her being here. It's a waste of money." I know I sound blunt, but I don't care. Mom can't afford to pay so much money to sleep the day away. What kind of life is that?

Diane smiles calmly and reassures me that Mom is still getting all of her meals and snacks, just at unusual times. "The kitchen is always open," she says. "Your mom can eat her meals in the middle of the night if she wants to."

Michelle says, "Your mom is eating well." She flips through a folder. "And her weight is stable."

Diane says that even though Mom misses some of the daytime social activities, she gets plenty of stimulation from the late afternoon and evening activities. She enjoys the crossword puzzle groups, and although Mom usually listens more than she offers the answers, she is "definitely paying attention and engaged." Diane says Mom is really good at the game in which they try to guess names from the past, and she's impressed that Mom knows some answers when no one else does. Mom also likes old movies.

Diane says that my mother particularly enjoys the company of one of the nighttime RAs, who sits with her in her room, looks at magazines with her, and talks to her. "The nighttime RA is extremely soft-spoken and gentle," she says, "and your mom seems to like that." She speculates that Mom may be staying up late because she sees that her favorite RA is there and wants to be with her.

"We believe in letting residents keep the schedule they prefer," Diane says. "We will not physically force your mom to get out of bed if she doesn't want to."

Diane's tone is calm, never defensive, and I begin to think that I could grow to respect this director. I begin to relax.

I mention how Mom's mouth is dry because of what I have assumed to be a reaction to her new incontinence medication. "It's hard for me as her daughter," I tell them slowly, struggling to find the right words, "to see one of the last things she still has—her speech—impaired because of a medication."

Michelle says that yes, this kind of incontinence medication can cause dry mouth. She frowns. "It's really too bad." She offers to call Dr. Claiborne and ask that my mom be taken off the medication.

Diane then suggests that Mom no longer needs an outside aide to help her with the transition. "We can provide her with everything she needs," she says.

I'm instantly skeptical. It sounds like a sales pitch. I doubt my mother will get all the stimulation she needs within these walls, and I intend to continue the private aides.

"Okay then," Diane says after a while. She sits up straighter and shifts to cross her legs the other way. "Now we should take a look at the care plan."

The care plan? I think, squinting and cocking my head to the side. What have we been doing for the past half hour if not the care plan? Clearly I don't know how these things work.

Diane and Michelle pick up pieces of paper (they don't offer me a copy) and Diane summarizes the services they will provide. She explains that, because of Mom's staying up until the early morning hours and her agitated state when she finally wakes up, there is a new charge of $288 a month for "reluctance to accept care." Those services include "verbal or physical assistance" and "a second person to provide assistance."

"So," I ask, "it costs Mom more to be up half the night?"

"Not that much more," Diane says, and offers an apologetic half smile.

I frown but say nothing. She continues: "There is an additional $180 assessed for this first thirty-day period for 'assistance managing behaviors when demonstrating anxious, disruptive or obsessive behavior requiring additional attention.' " She doesn't really explain what this means, or give examples, just says it's minor and probably part of the whole sleep/rest disruption; it may work itself out. But there is no time to ask for examples as I can sense they are winding things up.

The fees for Mom's first month of personal care (on top of the basic charges), Diane tells me, come to $1,440. Due to a complicated arrangement with their parent company and New York State, Elm Haven will deduct $430 each month from that fee. Unlike many other assisted living facilities, Elm Haven already includes in their basic charges a fee for some medical and personal care; they subtract this amount to avoid duplicate fees. Thus Mom's personal care plan will cost $1,010 a month, bringing her total monthly bill to about $4,800.

I'm sure I look shocked. This charge for personal care is twice what they estimated during the initial interview. Diane reassures me that I can request a care plan meeting at any time to go over what services and charges are necessary. She points out that Mom's "grade" on the assessment for each category of care is an A or a B, with D being the highest level of care, which means, she says, that Mom is doing quite well. She asks me to sign the Resident Assessment Summary Report and goes out to make me a copy.

Michelle kneels down in front of my chair and makes a joke—I don't remember what—"just to get you to smile, Martha."

As I walk down the hall in a daze with Michelle I ask how often the residents are taken out of the building to special events. If I discontinue Maggie's aide to save money, I think to myself, I don't want Mom inside all the time except when I take her out. Michelle doesn't say "once or twice a week" or anything concrete like that, but suggests I take a look at the calendar, and asks me if I get one in the mail (I don't). In the activities director's office she hands me a copy. I can tell at a glance that the outside ("OS") activities are few and far between. Michelle points out a concert in the living room that night that she thinks my mom will enjoy. Again I suspect that my mother needs more outside activities than Elm Haven will provide.

I find Mom sitting in a rocking chair in the living room. Michelle puts some music from the forties on the CD player, and Diane sits next to a woman and talks with her. The woman, with short gray hair and far-away eyes, says to Diane, "I don't like you."

"Well," Diane says, "I like *you.*" She asks the woman if she can give her a hug. A moment later Diane and the woman are standing up, holding hands, dancing. Other residents clap along to the music.

I whisper in Mom's ear that I want to go to her room to check her bra size. I need to order her some new bras.

"Mine are a little…worn out, are they?" she whispers back, enjoying our game.

I tell her I will be right back, and lope off to her room where I find only one bra in her drawer and the size is rubbed off the tag. I decide to wait until my next visit to check the bra she's wearing.

It's an hour past when I thought I would be done with the meeting, and I am eager to get home to Morgan, who's still in elementary school and arrives home before Andrew, a middle-schooler. I also want an excuse to leave, to get back to my own life. I did what I came to do.

Violent Behavior

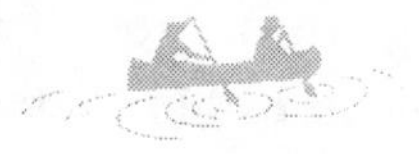

A few days later, at eight-thirty at night, I get a call from Elm Haven.

"There was an incident with your mom tonight that I need to let you know about," an RA says.

"Is my mom okay?" I interrupt, panic rising.

"Yes, she's okay," she says, though she sounds shaken. She tells me that they could not find Mom, looked everywhere for her, then finally found her in another resident's empty room where she was half undressed and getting into bed. The RA "redirected" her to get dressed and go back to her own room. As the RA was helping her pull her pants up, Mom reached down, grabbed the pen the woman had in her pocket and tried to stab the pen into the woman's neck.

"Luckily the pen was closed. It just left a red mark on her neck," this RA tells me now. The RA had reached for the emergency cord by the bed, and when two other RAs rushed in they found them standing stock still, Mom still pressing the pen to the RA's neck.

I can't wrap my mind around the idea that Mom tried to stab someone in the neck with a pen. I can see the steely look in her eye, but she's never been violent. This is new. I don't understand it.

The RA tells me that they had to call me to report it and they must send an incident report to Mom's doctor, too. I feel awful for the night RA, and ask if there is anything that I should do or can do, and the RA on the phone says no. I don't think to ask if the night RA was my mom's favorite or perhaps someone new.

Ben is with me in our living room when I get the call. I'm shaking inside as I tell him what happened. He gives me a long hug. A half hour later I start to have a panic attack—the first in several years. My back heats up; I feel warmth and pressure in my chest, and I'm agitated. When this happened before, well before Mom moved in, I went to the emergency room no less than five times, scared I was having a heart attack. It was diagnosed as either a panic attack or an allergic reaction to something, no one was sure. I am sensitive to wheat, and had wheat this evening. Now I ask Ben to find one of my old medications for anxiety. I take a half dose and feel better within minutes. I pat the couch so Ben will sit next to me and he holds me in his arms.

First thing in the morning, even before I brew my coffee or take a shower, I sit at my desk and skim the book *The 36-Hour Day* for information about dementia and violent behavior. I read that "combativeness" is common in later stages if the person feels threatened or stressed, but I can find no examples of people trying to plunge sharp instruments into other people's necks—just biting, slapping, kicking, that kind of thing. What Mom did last night seems to me to be more homicidal, more evil. At the moment I want nothing to do with her. If I thought it was purely the dementia I would feel sorry for her. But that anger is too much like her anger when she was anxious and kicked me out of the house.

I'm afraid that whatever is left of that anxiety buried deep inside her will make her more prone to dangerous acts of violence now that any inhibitions are gone.

I search online for "Alzheimer's disease, violence" and find nothing like "my mother tried to stab an aide."

I wish the Alzheimer's caregivers support group was meeting the following Tuesday, but it will be in a few more weeks. I consider calling Dan, the facilitator.

As it's a weekend, Diane, the director at Elm Haven, returns my call from her home. Does this kind of thing happen often? I ask. Diane says no, it's the first time something like this has happened. Wow, I think. Mom is a freak, a nut job who's dangerous to others. But, Diane says, she talked to the RA and the RA is fine and Mom is back to her old self, "sitting happily in the library, her eyes that bright blue."

Diane tells me that before Mom grabbed the pen she was not acting agitated, but she did say to the RA something like, "This is my space—get out of my space." Diane tells me as well that my mother might have the stomach flu that's going around and that's why she acted out as she did. They will just keep an eye on her and I shouldn't worry. "Feel free to call me at home," she says.

I'm beginning to see that Diane really might be open to talking to family members as a social worker or counselor, that's she not just saying it.

In the afternoon I call Maggie and ask her if the private aide, Candy, could take Mom out to only one place, for a maximum of three hours, rather than to two or three places for six hours, as she has done a few times. I tell her about Mom's incident Friday night after she was out with Candy, and how I was told that at dinner Mom was agitated, talking on and on about "that bitch." I tell her I'm not assuming that there is a correlation between her time with

Candy that day and her violence later that night, but I want her to know that my experience with Mom, even before the dementia, is that she may seem to be having a good time in the daytime but will get burned out if there is too much going on. She'll turn against people in the evening, wanting only to be left alone. Her brain seems to go on overload.

Maggie listens patiently and agrees to limit Mom's outings to one or two destinations, no more than three hours, no problem. Then quietly she asks me how I'm doing. I feel grateful, again, that someone asks me that.

"I just can't understand what happened. Have you ever heard of something like that?"

"Sure, that kind of thing can happen, especially if the person is afraid. In your mom's mind she could have been defending herself. She might have felt cornered."

I tell her what Diane said about Mom saying, "This is my space, get out of my space."

"The girls," Maggie says, meaning the Elm Haven RAs, "should have known that if your mother felt scared or angry or said anything like 'get out of my space' that they should have backed off and left her alone for a few minutes." She sounds more upset with how the RAs acted than with Mom's behavior.

For the first time since Friday, I feel less ashamed of Mom, less afraid that what she did was abnormal even for people with dementia. I feel as if it's going to be all right.

An Evening to Remember

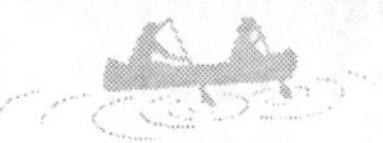

Thanksgiving morning Morgan wakes up with the stomach flu and throws up every half hour. I have a mild case of bronchitis again and struggle to make two pumpkin pies and one banana cream pie as Ben starts the turkey, stuffing, and cranberry sauce. At mid-day I decide that, even if it's a holiday, it's just a really bad day to have my mother over for a meal. As Mom used to say in her 12-step program, "Remember that a holiday is just another day. There's no need to get stressed out trying to make it perfect."

Surprisingly, I feel no guilt. I assume that Mom will not remember what day it is, even if the staff serves her turkey and pie. She may appreciate the idea of Thanksgiving for a moment, but then the thought will be gone.

A week later I take Mom out on a Friday night to hear the Vienna Boys' Choir perform at a theater downtown. She has always appreciated classical music and I know she will love this concert, but

I dread the whole process of getting Mom to the theater on time. I called Elm Haven to tell them when I'd pick her up, but when I arrive she still needs to be taken to the bathroom. When I finally get her in the car, I remind myself that if we miss the concert, I could just take her out for ice cream and bring her home. But—darn it—I really want her to be able to enjoy this performance. Most likely she will never have another chance to hear the Vienna Boys' Choir in person. I have to get her there, I think.

We make it with a few moments to spare. Throughout the concert Mom sits quietly; she knows how to be a good audience member. When I was in middle and high school, Mom would drive an hour in order that the two of us could hear the Rochester Philharmonic. Her knowledge of how to listen quietly without disturbing the performers or other audience members must lie embedded in the deepest parts of her mind; she doesn't talk to me or squirm; with her legs crossed, her hands folded in her lap, and her chin tilted up a bit, Mom gazes at the stage and smiles.

After the concert, as we walk past the stores decorated for the holidays, Mom turns to me and says, "I want you to know…that I just love this—tonight, being with you."

I say, "Me, too, Mom," though I'm not sure what she means. What I hear is not "being with you," but "tonight." I want to believe that what she loved the most was the concert. I want to give her these kinds of experiences. What I'm not quite ready to give her each time we see each other is the more intimate gift of my sustained attention, my presence, my self.

Back at Elm Haven, Mom shines, exuberant. "I had a *wonderful* time," she tells the RAs. I'm surprised that she remembers where we were, but she seems to know that we just heard a choir. She lies on top of her bed, and when I kiss her goodbye she's still smiling; her joy nearly lifts her off the bedcovers.

• • •

The next day, after cleaning the cottage, I arrive at Elm Haven for their holiday tea party. An RA tells me right away how much fun my mother had the night before, how much she talked about it. Michelle, the nurse, and Crystal, the sales director, come over to chat with Mom and say hi to me as we sit in the dining room, and they tell me again how happy Mom was when she got home last night from the concert.

Michelle adds, "You know, we love your mom. We just think she's a sweetheart." To Mom, she says, "I could just squeeze you!"

"You can squeeze me...all you want!" Mom replies.

Diane, the director, tells me, "Your mom seems happy here. I think she feels safe."

I believe her. I no longer suspect the friendliness of the staff to be fake. They genuinely enjoy the residents and their jobs, and I believe my mother can tell.

Reckoning

In late December, when I go over Mom's bills, I feel nauseated. I have been putting off figuring out how long her savings will keep her at Elm Haven, not wanting to know. I finally sit down with a calculator. She has $7,000 left in her checking account, $55,500 in mutual funds, and $33,000 in her IRA. She has the same incidental expenses as she had at Greenway, such as Medicare premiums and supplemental insurance, with the exception that she now pays $160 a month for Depends. After tapping in all the figures, I estimate that my mother will be able to afford Elm Haven for an additional twenty-one months. That's longer than I expected, but still not enough time. At seventy-five, she is young and could live many more years with dementia.

I'm beginning to like the staff at Elm Haven so much that I want to keep her here as long as possible. I consider selling the cottage to pay for her care. I think about how it's been in the family for three generations, and how renting it in the summer will, over ten years or so, equal the amount we would earn in a sale. I think about how Mom might get injured and have to go to a nursing home anyway. She might die unexpectedly before we spend all the proceeds from a sale. The more I ruminate, the more I believe she would not want me to sell it.

In 2007 in New York State, she'll qualify for Medicaid as soon as she spends down her assets to less than $4,200. She transferred the cottage to me in the spring of 2005, and at that time the state had a "look back" period, in which they check for transfers and gifts of assets, of only three years. (It has now been extended to five years, but Mom is exempt because the transfer happened before the law changed.) If we apply for her Medicaid after the spring of 2008, the value of the cottage would not count as an asset. I lean toward keeping the cottage for our children, as their Grammy would want.

I fear what will come next. To avoid a nursing home, I call Dan at the Office for the Aging to find out if there are any assisted living places in our county that accept Medicaid. He tells me that there are three Medicaid-funded assisted living places within a forty-five-minute drive of our city, but they are not "secure" for people who wander, and they will not accept people who need the level of care that Mom requires.

It makes no sense to me that Medicaid in our state pays for nursing home care for people with dementia, but usually not "secure" memory care assisted living such as Elm Haven, which costs, on average nationwide, about thirty percent less than a nursing home with dementia care. In 2011 the national average for dementia care in a semi-private nursing home room will be $222 per day, or $81,030 a year; assisted living with dementia care will average $152 per day, or $55,428 per year. I suspect that our government counts on the fact that most adult children fear nursing homes, and our own guilt for considering one, and that we will choose instead to pay out of our pockets for a private facility or care for our parents at home, saving the state billions of dollars a year.

Dan suggests I call the county's Long-term Care Services office, the department that finds institutional care for people who do not have private funds, and they tell me the same thing, that the next step in our area can only be a nursing home. I make a note to visit a few nursing homes over the next year.

Compared to her last six months in assisted living, Mom's first six months in memory care are extraordinarily peaceful and healthy. She doesn't fall. And now that she's taking a melatonin supplement, as Michelle, the head nurse, suggested to regulate her sleep cycle, Mom's going to bed and getting up at normal hours, eating breakfast and joining the morning activities.

To stretch her savings, I've canceled the private aide through Maggie's agency. I tell Maggie on the phone that I'm trying to save money in case Mom needs a private aide for medical reasons. I tell her how very grateful I feel for her help and reassurance.

It's February and I'm asleep in Ben's old room at his parents' house in Queens. We're visiting for Chinese New Year, the first time we've been out of town since our vacation in August. Twice in the night I sit up, jolted out of deep sleep. "Where is Mom? Is she okay?" I ask myself. For a moment I can't remember if she's back at our house, wandering around alone, or in bed in her old room at Greenway, uncovered, cold. Then I see her; she's in the living room at Elm Haven next to the fireplace, and in the dining room chatting with her friends. She's hundreds of miles away from me but she is safe and loved. She's fine. I take a breath, close my eyes, and fall back to my own dreams.

Sex and Dementia

In early April of 2008, I cash out the last of Mom's mutual funds in one fell swoop, $52,500, and deposit them in her checking account. Only her IRA remains—$33,700. Each closing of an account sounds to me like a death knell.

Then, a new shock.

I get a call from Michelle, the nurse, on a Saturday afternoon. My mother has been in Elm Haven for seven months.

"Martha, your mom is fine but I need to tell you that we found her in bed with another resident. We found her with Bill." She pauses. "Our rule is that she has to go to the emergency room to be checked for trauma. She seems fine, but if you can't take her, one of us will have to take her."

I've met Bill, a short, portly, balding man with a walker. I've seen Mom cozied up next to him on the couch, her eyes shining.

"Are you sure she has to go? What if I say, as her health care proxy, that I don't think she needs to go?" I'm not at all surprised that the staff found Mom in bed with a man. I know that my mother is a sexual being. Over the years she's mentioned her attraction to this man and that. Whatever Mom and Bill were doing was as consensual as sex can be for two people unable to make and remember decisions. And I bet Bill isn't required to go to the E.R.

"It's just a precaution," Michelle says. "We have to make sure she's not injured."

"Fine. I'll be right there." I'd rather take Mom myself than have an RA take her—I can keep her calm and unafraid, and she might be there for hours.

On my way to the car, I see my neighbor, Karen, one of the facilitators of our village discussion of dementia, the one who works with caregivers and whose father had early-onset Alzheimer's disease. I tell her my mother was found in bed with a man.

"Yes!" Karen says. She smiles and gives me a thumbs-up.

I ask her if her father in the later stages of Alzheimer's ever climbed in bed with a woman other than his wife.

"All the time!" she says. "It happened all the time."

I tell her that I'm fine with it, I just don't want Mom dragged to the E.R. each time it happens.

"I know. It's crazy, isn't it?" she says. She shakes her head, then reaches to give me a hug.

At Elm Haven, I find Mom perky and smiling, sitting in the main living room. Her hair is a bit disheveled. The two RAs who meet me are calm but their eyes are serious, their brows furrowed.

"I'm sorry I couldn't clean your mom up," one says. "She had a bowel movement, but..."—her voice trails off—"I don't think we're supposed to clean her up...in case there's evidence or something."

I nod. She hands me a pile of clean clothes for Mom in case I change her at the hospital. "They might need the Depends we found her in, for evidence, too," she says. "It's dirty, though." She frowns again.

"I guess we should bring it," I say. "I don't know how these things work." They seem to be looking to me to know what to do, but they might have more experience than I do with this sort of thing.

One asks me if I want to press charges. "We have to ask you that," she says.

I tell her no, I don't, and shake my head. "I think this kind of thing is completely normal. And Mom seems fine."

I would expect my mother to initiate cuddling in bed, or more. And I hope the staff treats these incidents as normal and not a cause of upset.

Mom walks to the car with me without signs of injury or emotional trauma. On the two-minute drive to the hospital Mom wants to untie the plastic bag with the dirty Depends to see what's inside, and she won't stop when I ask her. I snap at her for the first time in a long time—"Mom, let go!" She holds on tight but I manage finally to snatch it away. I take a deep breath and will myself to start over. My plan is to treat this E.R. exam as just another doctor's visit, to take the next few hours one minute at a time. Mom probably won't realize she's in the hospital; she'll believe she's just in a doctor's office. I plan to squeeze her hand and enjoy her company, even if in between we have to deal with nurses and doctors and a possible exam of Mom's private parts. If we're required to go through this, I might as well make it as pleasant as possible for both of us, just another outing.

The nursing staff treats Mom gently, never asking what happened or too many questions that she can't answer. I tell her main nurse, right away, just as I did with the aides at Elm Haven, "I want you to know that I'm not worried about this. I think it's entirely natural." I don't know why I think it's important to say this, but I do. The nurse looks puzzled and says nothing.

A woman in street clothes with a nametag comes in and asks to speak with me in the hallway. She's the crisis counselor, she explains, and gently asks me if I think a complete exam is necessary. I say no, and she agrees. A nurse will simply do an external, visual exam to check for bruising.

As Mom and I wait for a doctor to check in, we share a pint of blueberries I brought from the store, and I hand her a can of raspberry spritzer to sip. I've learned to be prepared for long hours in the E.R. I brought a newspaper and a book to read, and took a few extra minutes to drive out of my way to pick up the snacks and food for dinner for the two of us in case we were there through dinner time. I'm no longer willing to leave my mother alone in the E.R., even for a few minutes, to get food from the cafeteria.

I hold my mother's hand through the nurse's exam, which shows no bruising. When the nurse cleans Mom, I feel embarrassed for Mom, but she just smiles at me and squeezes my hand. Afterward, sitting up, Mom says, "I feel a bit sore" and points toward her tailbone. I wonder for the first time if perhaps she fractured a bone again, if Bill was on top of her, pressing down. The last thing she needs is another fracture. Or maybe the padded discs in her HipSavers pressed against her bottom and left a sore spot. A doctor asks Mom to sit all the way up and he gently presses here and there; finding no pain, he pronounces her fine. I wonder if he'll order an X-ray, but he doesn't. I decide to wait and see how she feels later; she's been through enough.

While we wait for her discharge papers, Mom rolls over under the blanket, smiles at me again, and closes her eyes. "I'll be right here, Mom," I say. As she sleeps I hold her hand and stroke her hair, gossamer between my fingers and her tender forehead. My fingertips skim her temple in gentle arcs; I touch the tracings of veins and pulse, her skin as light and thin as phyllo.

• • •

When we arrive back at Elm Haven three RAs hug Mom tight. Mom kisses each of them on the cheek. From across the living room where she's leading a discussion, Vicki, the activities director, cries, "Look who's here! Welcome back, Judy!"

"Thank you!" Mom says. "It's good...to be here!"

After I kiss Mom goodbye, an RA gently turns her away from the door, her arm around Mom's waist, with promises of soup and dinner. I leave without worry, confident that the staff will give my mother lots of extra attention. From my car I call Diane to update her as I promised I would. I ask her to have the staff keep an eye on Mom's discomfort around her pelvis. I'm calm. Through a potentially upsetting and confusing experience, I managed to help my mother feel peaceful. I fully accept, as well, that I am my mother's advocate in all situations, that I am the one person who knows best what my mother needs and wants. I no longer shirk or swerve or defer.

I do feel nervous, though, about one thing—talking with Diane about their policies around residents and sex. I postpone it. I fear that, if I ask her to clarify their policies, she'll resent my asking. Do they have written guidelines for monitoring sexual encounters between residents for safety, privacy and consent? What if they don't have a policy? What if they do, but it's too strict and Mom and Bill are kept apart?

Two weeks after the incident I gather my courage after a visit with Mom, pull myself into Diane's office, and plant myself in a chair by her desk. I explain that I'd like my mother to have enough privacy to enjoy Bill's company but enough supervision to make sure that she's not being forced to do something she doesn't want to do.

Diane nods, leans back in her chair, looks at me pensively through her glasses, and smiles. "We all love to have someone to crawl into bed with," she says.

"So why did Mom have to be seen in the E.R.?" I ask. "Is it a state rule?"

"Not exactly," Diane says. "Whenever there is physical contact between residents, we're required by the state to offer both a police report and a physical health assessment.

"If I had been here when it happened," she continues, "I could have asked your mom if she'd let me check for bruising or other injury. But residents don't expect us to treat them like we're doctors. They don't expect us to check them in that way. They might be more comfortable with a doctor in the hospital."

"That makes sense," I say. "And Mom did have some discomfort around her hips."

"Right."

I tell her I noticed that the last few times I'd visited, since the incident, Bill always has a private aide in the same room with him.

"Yes, he will have an aide with him twenty-four hours a day. We can't have him approaching the women here for sex. Even if your mother was not traumatized, even if she welcomed it, other women may not. They may have never been married, may have a different sexual orientation, or may not want to be touched. We just can't take a chance."

"Of course." But if Bill's family has to pay for a private aide, I think to myself, that's an awfully high price for them to keep him at Elm Haven. If the women have to go to the E.R. after a sexual encounter, but not the men, the families of the men are penalized in turn by having to pay for extra supervision—as if the men are always the perpetrators and the women victims. The idea galls me, a child of the seventies and young woman of the eighties. I assume a woman's needs to be equal to a man's.

"You see," Diane continues, "Bill likes about six of the women here. That's common in men with Alzheimer's disease. And it's common with women, too—that loss of inhibition." She pauses. "I do know that Bill can't perform. I found that out from his wife after the incident. She lives right down the road, and told me he can't do anything. Even so, we have to be very careful. With your mom, as you pointed out the other day, we have to think about brittle bones and possible injury."

"That reminds me," I say. "I never found out exactly what Mom and Bill were doing when they were discovered together. I should probably know the details, you know, for medical reasons."

"We're not sure what they were up to. Your mom was sitting on the edge of Bill's bed with her shirt on but her pants off. She was still wearing her HipSavers and Depends. Bill had his pants and underwear off and was standing in front of her. It wasn't clear if they were just getting into bed, just getting out, or doing something else."

I tell Diane that I understand that Elm Haven must do what is easiest and safest for everyone, but I hope that Mom will be allowed to sit next to Bill, maybe snuggle with him, in a common room, supervised. I know she still notices him. Mom and I walked past him today as he was sitting in the TV room outside Mom's bedroom and she paused to smile and wiggle her fingers at him. He gave her a big smile and waved back.

"Yes, she still has eyes for him," Diane says. "She can certainly spend time with him. He just has to have an aide with him."

I know that Mom has already lost most of her autonomy, but I leave disappointed for her nevertheless, saddened that she's now lost this new source of comfort and the sparkle in her eye.

Sharp And Sweet

During this first year at Elm Haven, Mom moves from Stage Five of mid-stage Alzheimer's disease to Stage Six: severe cognitive decline, or late mid-stage Alzheimer's. I don't recognize the new stage when it happens, but looking back, I can see it: her difficulty remembering her personal history; the lack of awareness of recent events and her surroundings; needing help with dressing; the sleep disturbances; needing full assistance in the bathroom; and the incontinence of bladder and bowel. Unlike many people living with Stage Six Alzheimer's disease, though, she has not shown signs of daily paranoia, or of compulsive behavior such as hand wringing.

Also typical of Stage Six, Mom seems to clearly recognize familiar faces, including mine, but she can no longer name us. I don't mind. I can tell by the way she smiles at me and reaches for me, by that deep, particular twinkle in her eye, that she recognizes me as her daughter. That makes me happy.

* * *

I learn that Carrie, our favorite RA, has "moved on." She was such a sociable person; I imagine she grew bored with her promotion to full-time medication cart attendant. I doubt she enjoyed having to peer at the tiny notations in the medication logs and dispense pills all day.

Her departure reminds me again of Lauren Kessler's book *Dancing with Rose*, in which she chronicles working for three months as an RA in a memory care facility. Turnover is so frequent, she says, that "a year is a long time in the life of an RA." Without a nursing degree, personable RAs usually find little room in elder care for advancement, a pay raise, or respect.

I'll miss Carrie, but I'm relieved that the young woman replacing her seems equally bright-eyed and thorough. I hope this one sticks around.

I've finally come to appreciate the difficulty of the RA's job, and I accept that if small things do not get done—if Mom's shirt has a stain, or her teeth look fuzzy as if they weren't brushed well, or at all, that morning—I cannot expect the staff to be perfect, as I cannot expect myself to be perfect. This is a hard lesson for me, perfectionist that I am.

I try to be the kind of family member who helps the staff rather than expecting to be waited on. At parties and holiday gatherings, I don latex gloves, stand at the kitchen counter, and help the staff dish the food. One weekend I spend two full days helping Vickie, the activities director, create an album with photos showing the residents dancing and batting balloons around the living room, planting flowers and playing badminton in the courtyard, snapping Vickie's home-grown green beans in the dining room, and trying on Halloween wigs at the mall.

Thanks to dementia, I've learned to not sweat the small stuff—and much of what happens to my mother is small stuff. I don't worry when an RA calls me to tell me that Mom is upset because another resident hit her on the head with a doll. Or when we move Mom to a double room to save her money, and she gets a bloody nose from a scuffle with her new roommate (who is soon moved to a different room). As my mother forgets, I relax. These incidents fall from my mother's memory, and mine, like used stamps from paper.

There is one thing that bothers me, though. I'm ashamed that my mother has started to play with her feces. Michelle the head nurse tells me that Mom seems fascinated with their texture. A few other residents do that, too, Michelle says. There's even a name for it: scatolia. I'm embarrassed by her behavior, but more ashamed of myself because I'm relieved beyond words that I don't have to clean her. At a care plan meeting I try to joke that the $250 a month Elm Haven has continued to charge Mom for needing extra attention at night, even though she's now sleeping on a normal schedule, is "well worth" their extra work. I can't imagine doing this.

When I visit I find myself glancing at my mother's fingernails as I hold her hand; they're always clean. The staff keeps her fingernails trimmed short. They tell me that during the day they take her to the bathroom every two hours, and at night check her hourly.

Once I take a furtive glance at her fingers I'm able to push these ugly images from my mind. Perhaps I'm "in the moment," perhaps in denial; either way, I hold onto the mother I know.

Grape pie is a local specialty along the shores of Silver Lake. My mother and I often enjoyed my great-aunt's pie from the Concord grapes in her side yard. When I made a grape pie for Ben and the kids in early October and brought a piece to Mom, the RAs had never heard of grape pie and thought it was blueberry. That's when inspiration hit. To celebrate the one-year anniversary of Mom moving into Elm Haven, I decide to bake thirty-two grape pies, one for each of the Elm Haven staff members: the day shift, the night shift, the three nurses, the director and assistant, the maintenance guy, the cleaners, the kitchen crew.

For two days in my neighborhood's main dining room I pinch the skins off twenty-four quarts of purple grapes. I boil, then press the green pulp with a wooden spoon through a colander to separate the big, tooth-cracking seeds. I mix the skins, pulp and sugar into a crimson sauce, and roll out the store-bought crust. Andrew and Morgan help for a few hours with the skinning, and Morgan helps me deliver the pies in our van along with some of her home-baked lemon cookies. I tuck beneath the plastic wrap on each pie a photocopy of a thank-you note. We deliver the pies at night, and they fill every available counter and shelf in the kitchen. The maintenance man, I hear, eats two. Diane, the director, says they have never received such a special thank-you.

I don't regret the effort of making those pies, but I found out from a neighbor passing by, as I was ladling the pulp and skins into the crusts, that I didn't have to peel the grapes and separate the seeds after all. Concord grapes come in a seedless variety. Who knew? I was going by an old recipe, out-of-date.

I'm convinced that baking thirty-two grape pies is like caring for a parent with dementia. The reward is singular, both sharp and sweet—like bronzed, bare, late-autumn vines warmed by the lingering breezes of a deep, wide lake.

And if you aren't lucky enough as a caregiver to get the right advice at the right time, the job becomes much harder than it needs to be.

Financial Disaster

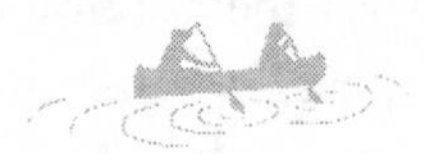

With the stock market crash in the autumn of 2008, the value of my mother's modest IRA falls from $33,000 in the summer to $22,500 in November. Now I watch the market more closely, prepared to withdraw the rest of her IRA at any moment.

At the end of October, on the day after my forty-fourth birthday, I realize that I haven't mentioned my birthday to my mother. I didn't even call her as I did the previous year. I no longer need her to show me she loves me in her old ways, to hold up to me, like a mirror, her enduring vision of me as a lovely and capable woman. Her smile, when I see her, is enough.

The holidays get easier and easier as well. Christmas Day, we lounge around as a family, Ben and I and the kids, and I feel no guilt for waiting to see Mom the next day. I no longer worry about finding just the right gifts for her, no longer feel disappointed if she doesn't coo over my choices. This year, my presents to her are simple: three blouses in her favorite colors, a box of chocolates, and our company. Mom sits in our living room and watches Andrew and Morgan play their new video games; she gazes at the old-fashioned, colored bulbs on our Fraser fir; she pets Trinka, now thirteen years old and blind and deaf, in her lap. While Ben prepares lunch, I sit in the chair next to Mom and we listen to the classical music CDs Ben gave me for Christmas. After lunch, the two of us look at photo albums; she still enjoys reading the captions. When I offer her our homemade, frosted Christmas cookies, shaped as a Santa and a wreath, and I say, "These are the same kind of cookies you used to make with me each year, Mom, all the time I was growing up," she's content to believe me.

I rise to take her home. Mom strolls across the room to her grandchildren, cups each of their faces in turn in her palms, smiles up at them, these towering grandchildren, and illuminates their eyes with hers. "I love you," she says.

In December and January I withdraw the remaining funds in her IRA. Her checking account now has enough for her to live at Elm Haven for ten more months.

She will soon qualify for Medicaid. With changes in New York State Medicaid law, in 2009 Mom will be allowed to keep more of her assets—$13,800, compared to $4,200 in 2007. I would need to start the application process in a few months, and find a nursing home.

Instead, I decide to sell the cottage. I'd rather say goodbye to the cottage where I spent summers as a child, where I'd hoped my children would bring their children, than see my mother leave the staff at Elm Haven.

In any case, Ben and the kids don't seem as attached to the cottage and the lake as I am. It's time to let it go. I'll split the proceeds of the sale between my mother's care and our children's college fund. I believe that's what she would want.

What If's

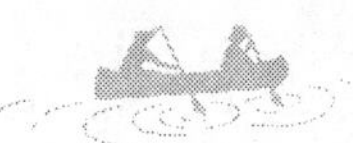

I realize that I haven't seen Henry in awhile, the handsome resident with the thick, salt-and-pepper hair who shuffled into Mom's room when she first arrived. One Saturday, as I help Vickie, the activities director, finish another photo album, I see Henry in the pictures, smiling at the camera.

Vickie joins me, harried but as upbeat as always, between shoveling the sidewalk and dealing with a sewer emergency. (On weekends there's no maintenance staff; as the administrator on duty she has to handle everything.) A young grandmother close to my age, tall and heavyset with long brown hair, she grows so attached to the residents that when they have to leave she visits them in their new facilities and has a hard time keeping to herself her opinion about where they "end up."

When I ask about Henry she takes a breath and says, "Yes, he's no longer here." She pauses. "He needed intensive care."

"He was a sweetheart," I say, and she agrees, her eyes sad. I want to ask her what happened to him, what kind of care he needed, but I don't.

Vickie points to another picture in which two women nap together on the living room couch, their heads touching. "And she's passed away," Vickie says, touching her finger to the woman on the left, a resident I don't remember.

"You get so attached," she says, and I nod.

In the pile of photos for the album I find two of my mother: She's sitting in the living room, listening to a band playing acoustic guitars. She looks unbelievably thin, with an almost ethereal expression on her face, her eyes half closed, her mouth curved in a smile.

I see not only her luminous presence, her enduring self, but something vulnerable, fading, closer than I would like to admit to the frailty I see in the faces of Henry and the woman who died. I realize that even though I've worked hard to make sure my mother enjoys the quality of her day-to-day life, I need to think more about her wishes for the end of her life. That stage may arrive more quickly than I anticipate.

Mothering my mother, I realize now, is not just about doing things, giving her things, or even about being there. It's also about facing head-on the larger "what if's."

When I meet with Diane, the director, and Michelle, the head nurse, for another care plan meeting, I remind them that my mother is Do Not Resuscitate, and ask that, if they dial 911 for my mother, they call me immediately. I don't want an ambulance crew doing anything to my mother that she wouldn't have wanted.

Diane and Michelle promise to call, of course, but they seem uncomfortable; they merely suggest that I make sure that I've given them New York State's "Non-Hospital Order Not to Resuscitate

(DNR)" form, signed by her doctor, which I have. I leave unsatisfied, worried in an abstract kind of way.

A few weeks later I read in the *New York Times* about a new advance-directive form available only in New York State from an insurance company, bright pink to catch the attention of ambulance crews. Called the MOLST form ("Medical Orders for Life-Sustaining Treatment"), it's been available since the previous summer but I hadn't heard about it. I order the form and the supplemental version for people who no longer have the capacity to consent, and schedule an appointment alone with Dr. Claiborne, Mom's doctor, to fill it out and get it signed.

I'm nervous that Dr. Claiborne may never have seen these forms before and will refuse to sign them. I'm nervous that she will object that I haven't brought my mother along to the appointment. (I realize much later that Medicare might not even reimburse Dr. Claiborne for this "end of life" discussion.) I'm nervous that Dr. Claiborne will think I'm trying to kill off my mother before her time.

All my fears are unfounded. She listens quietly and respectfully. She says, "I haven't seen this particular form, but that's okay." We review each section together and she signs her initials: Resuscitation, no; hospitalization, yes, with the following restrictions: feeding tube, no; intubation, no; antibiotics—yes (but not if Mom has something like pneumonia over and over, I say, if she's miserable and it's only antibiotics keeping her alive.) "Yes, we can revisit this form if we need to," the doctor says.

She looks up and squints softly at me over her bifocals. "At some point," she says, "your mom's quality of life may be so poor you won't even want her to *go* to the hospital."

"You're right. You're absolutely right." I smile, relieved that she's said what I was too nervous to suggest.

What Remains

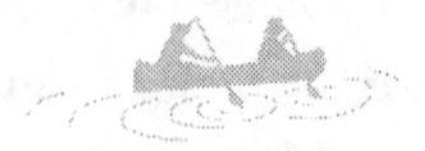

By August of 2009 the cottage is gone, sold to a lovely young couple who say they look forward to passing it on to their small daughter when she's grown.

Ben and I visit the cottage one last time alone. I gather a few personal items—my grandmother's silver salt and pepper shakers, the framed watercolors Mom painted years ago, the large picture of white sailboats leaning over the rolling waves of a blue-green lake. The new owners will be renting out the cottage, too, and everything else must stay as part of the sale: the furniture, the green wooden rowboat, and the contents of the boathouse. Inside the cottage, I think about how I'll miss the sound of the wooden kitchen cupboards clicking shut, the squeak of the metal kitchen drawers, the creak of the steep, drop-down stairs, the rustle of the folding bedroom doors. In the boathouse, I cry; I can smell the familiar mustiness of the shale floor, the dampness of the old cupboards and tables that hold the ancient outboard motor, the fishing lures, the canoe paddles and life vests. I think of how, as a child, I used to sit cross-legged on the shale inside the open doors, next to my grandfather. He'd sit in a green metal chair beside me, smoking a cigarette, and together we'd wait, silent and still, for approaching storms; we'd see the lightning strike the cliffs across the lake, hear the thunder and the rain, then feel the cool air rush over us. Now I close the heavy wooden doors, click the padlock shut, and walk along the beach. With Ben at my side, I stand and look out over the water, so deep and wide and timeless.

When I turn and look at the cottage, I am certain for a moment that I see the faces of my grandfather and grandmother, and my two great-aunts who loved the lake; they're floating over the roof, under the maple trees on the cliff, saying good-bye.

In early August, the balance of my mother's checking account—the last remnant of her savings—is only $3,300. The cottage sale happens in the nick of time, and I deposit $100,000 of the proceeds into Mom's account. It will be easier to keep track of the bookkeeping if I continue to write all of the checks for her care from her checking account, rather than from my checkbook. In a few months I will learn that I've made a serious error.

Rita, our neighbor living with Alzheimer's disease, moves out of our community to another state, into an assisted-living memory care place similar to Elm Haven. Her children want her to be closer to them, and despite our dedicated neighbors who volunteered to spend time with Rita, the cost of providing twenty-four-hour home care aides had become prohibitive.

I hear through the grapevine that, like Mom, Rita does well in memory care and smiles and laughs with the staff. She seems happier there than in her old home.

Through these past few years Rita and my mother have followed the same slow transformation. Rita is no longer speaking, and over the past year my mother's ability to talk has lessened to the point where she's silent most of the time. When she does try to speak, she'll say one or two words at a time, so muddled and soft I often can't understand them.

Today I'm surprised when Mom speaks more clearly than she has for months. Her sentences run short but cogent and crisp. We sit together in the woods beside my neighborhood and listen to six of my neighbors play their bongos in a drum circle. It's a warm Sunday afternoon in mid-November. Mom sits on a folding metal chair, I on the leafy dirt beside her. For a half hour we just gaze at the sunlight filtering through the branches. We stroke each other's thumbs. When I bounce my thumb to the rhythm of the bongos Mom laughs and points to my hand. She lifts her chin and turns her face to watch the people in the circle, smiles, and closes her eyes. When she turns back to me I say, "Do you like this, Mom?"

She says, "Yes, I do!"

Later she turns her big, bright eyes to me, taps the fingers of her right hand to her chest, and says, "I have...*feelings.*"

"You're happy?" I ask.

"Yes." She struggles a moment, then adds "Very!"

This is my first visit with her in a month as I've been sick with the flu. When I'm away for so long I don't know what I'll find. I think of what people always ask me when I tell them my mother has dementia: "Does she still know you?" I dread that my mother might look through me with no recognition.

I needn't have worried. In the living room at Elm Haven, she knew me the instant she saw me. She reached for me from her chair, throwing her arms up as if she was tossing a beach ball. "Hey!" she said. A year or two ago she might have said "Hey! There she is!" or "Hey, there's my girl!" but today it was just "Hey!" and the biggest smile in the world.

Here in the woods today I can feel my mother vibrant beside me. In this moment we fly back through the decades, past the harsh words we shared as mother and daughter, the slammed doors and tears and phone calls cut short—it's all gone. Nothing remains but the touch of her fingers to her chest and her smiling eyes.

As I'm cleaning our house I find the gray metal box in which Mom kept her "important papers," a fireproof container for her high school and college diplomas, her Social Security card, and a set of grades from college (all A's and B's). I squat on the bottom step of our stairs and open a small, white envelope marked "SAVE: Last letter from Mom." It's postmarked July 1976, to my mother from her mother, right before my grandmother died from a stroke at age sixty-five.

As soon as I read the envelope, I burst into tears. Mom adored her gentle, quiet mother, and lost her without warning. I cry for her loss, her pain. I cry, too, in gratitude that, at least for now, my mother and I still have each other.

In the box I also find my mother's two divorce decrees. The decree for my father, from Chiquaqua, Mexico, says little except that they were incompatible and had been separated for a year, but the one for my stepfather spills details of her life with him that I never knew. I could sense that he didn't care about me, but I never realized how unhappy my mother was with him. She rarely said anything bad about him, and they didn't fight in front of me. To me it has always seemed like she decided overnight to leave him. She shielded me from the worst of it.

I'd always thought Mom tolerated the rundown state of the old farmhouse, and have blamed her for tolerating it, thinking she was too weak-willed to demand better living conditions, but the divorce decree states that she fought with my stepfather for years to make repairs. It says that her income paid their bills while he spent his not on replacing the drywall on the exposed skeleton of the living room walls but on his hobbies—fishing and rifle shooting competitions. In addition to the bats, chipmunks, squirrels, and moles that I remember as living inside the house, there were also "spiders and rats." It lacked proper insulation, "plaster and wallpaper fell off the walls," and the heating system was "inadequate to heat the upstairs sleeping areas or the kitchen downstairs...Plaintiff became very emotionally distraught and depressed as a result of the defendant's refusal to provide adequate housing, and suffered from severe weight loss. Plaintiff had to take anti-depressant medication. Defendant has also acted in cruel and demeaning manner toward plaintiff and her minor daughter."

I think about the kinds of decisions I've been called to make, and will make, on behalf of my mother. I realize now that they mirror in intensity the decisions she made for my well being when I was a child. The major decisions of my mother's life that affected me the most—to divorce both my ill, abusive father and my neglectful, abusive stepfather, to support the two of us on her own, and to put herself into an alcoholism treatment program—were incredibly brave decisions that I have only now begun to appreciate.

Two and a half years after Mom's move to Elm Haven, they can no longer keep her well fed. She lost three pounds one week, and three the week before, down to one hundred and eleven pounds. Dr. Claiborne can find no medical explanation other than dementia. Mom's forgetting how to feed herself.

On a Saturday at the end of lunchtime I stop by to check on her. Everyone else is done with their meal but I find Mom sitting alone at the small "cueing" table where the RAs coach her through the steps of eating. (As they explained to me on the tour, Elm Haven cannot, lacking an "enriched" assisted living license, spoon the food into her mouth.) She's working her way through a bowl of ice cream, the one food she always remembers how to eat. A new RA I don't recognize tells me, "Lots of times your mom doesn't want us to talk to her. She looks away and ignores us. When she gets like that we just leave her alone."

That's wise, I think.

A year ago at my caregiver support group I learned that, to someone with dementia, a full plate with several foods crowded against each other can look unappealing and confusing. I started then to request that Mom be served her meals one dish and one utensil at a time, protein first. In addition to ice cream, she also gets high-fat meals and extra gravy. The chocolate liquid supplement she started drinking a few months ago gave her loose stools, so they switched to fortified juice three times a day. Each month Mom pays an extra $150 for the supplements and $120 on her personal care plan for the RAs to serve them to her.

Today it looks like the RAs followed my request to offer one food at a time, as I see the individual bowls off to the side, but they lie untouched.

I'd like nothing more than to deny it, but my mother is nearing the end of her stay in this lovely place. She's declining again, now one of Elm Haven's frailest residents.

Much later, I figure out that she is crossing the boundary of Stage Six to Stage Seven of Alzheimer's disease. In Stage Seven, "late-stage" Alzheimer's disease, the person cannot remember how to use a spoon or fork and needs to be spoon-fed. Swallowing becomes difficult, and they must be fed soft, then pureed food. Though they may retain the ability to say a few words, they lose the ability to have a conversation; their muscles grow rigid and they lose the ability to walk; they need help with every movement, every task; they may lose the ability to smile, sit without support, or hold up their head. Eventually they lie rigid in bed, nearly unresponsive. Stage Seven can last, I will learn, from several weeks to several years.

Part of me denies that my mother will end up like this, alive but stiff and unseeing. I cannot imagine it.

Honesty

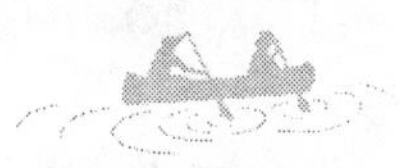

In February, I bundle Mom up for a short walk outside. It's cool but the sidewalks are bare of snow and the breeze is gentle. As usual, we leave her walker inside and I hold her arm. This past year she's walked very slowly, gingerly, as if she might crumble at any moment. I can hear her breathe beside me in short little puffs, just as she did when we climbed together up the hill at the cottage. She catches my eye and smiles.

So faint I almost don't hear her, she says, "You're nice."

"Thanks, Mom." I'm not sure what to say so I point past the bare branches of the trees. "Can you see the lake down there without your glasses?" (The glasses have long since disappeared. When Mom first moved into Elm Haven, Diane, the director, and I agreed that it made no sense to get Mom new glasses. She would just keep taking them off, or lose them.)

"Sure."

"See how it's frozen down on the end there?"

"Mm-hmm."

"Are you cold? You look cold."

Mom laughs and reaches her mittened hand for the scarf around her neck. I take that as a "yes" so turn us toward the door. I feel tears coming. I stop and face her. I take a deep breath and tell her I love her.

She crinkles a smile and looks deeper into my eyes.

"I know we've had our moments...you know, when we didn't get along." I pause, searching for recognition in her eyes. She squints slightly as if she's confused or worried. My tears flow faster now but she's quiet, watching me.

"I just want you to know...I just want to tell you...that I love you. I really love you." I squeeze her hand tighter. She smiles again but her eyes look serious.

"I know all the things you've done for me my whole life. And I want you to know how much you mean to me."

I want to say "Mom, do you understand?" but I don't.

She still studies me. What's going on under that concerned expression? I imagine that Mom can't remember the complexity of our history. I imagine that she's just trying to understand what in the world I'm talking about in this present moment. But I could be wrong.

When I say "I love you" again, her expression lightens. She reaches for both my hands and squeezes them. With that movement, that simple gesture, I know in my heart that my mother is telling me how special I am to her.

I ask for a hug. We hold each other for a long, sweet moment in the crisp, winter air.

Lately I've begun to wonder if I treat my mother too much like a child in the way I speak to her and the subjects I choose. In her book *Forget Memory: Creating Better Lives for People with Dementia*, Anne Davis Basting writes that "age stereotypes can yield patronizing behaviors like speaking in a high perky voice [and] talking only of simple subjects ('How about that weather!')..." I don't speak in a high voice, but I do try to be perky at all times. I purposely keep my banter light, as if Mom is losing, along with her language, her adult insight, wisdom and full range of emotion. In *Learning to Speak Alzheimer's*, Joanne Koenig Coste writes that we should "assume that the patient can still register feelings that matter." I have assumed that, beyond her steady love for me, Mom's other feelings have grown fewer, less frequent, and shallow.

John Zeisel writes in his book, *I'm Still Here: A Breakthrough Approach to Understanding Someone Living with Alzheimer's,* that when we communicate with a person living with dementia, "honesty means being yourself"—not shying away, as I so often have, from sharing my true feelings in fear that I'll upset my mother. He believes that a person living with dementia continues to grow in new ways, to develop new relationships and deepen old ones, and deserves to be treated as a whole, complicated, mature person.

If we are honest about our feelings around a person with dementia, he says, they "can do this honestly as well." Whether we're sad or happy, the person with dementia will feel "particularly good when he can express a feeling, whether of concern, empathy, fear, or love"—in words, if they still have their language, or with touch, gesture, or facial expressions.

Reading these three books this spring has made me consider for the first time that there's probably much more going on in my mother's mind than I've thought. With this realization I feel a deep regret and sadness. Two years ago, when Mom's words first became jumbled, when she became incontinent, when she stayed in the rehab center, I treated her as if she was no longer here, as if her brain were so diminished she would be unable to feel lonely, lost, or scared. When she said things in the rehab center such as

"Martha, how did you know I was here?" and looked close to tears, I assumed she was just confused.

Maybe I avoided her true feelings because it would have been too painful for both of us, and I couldn't do anything about them beyond visiting her nearly every day as I did. In fact, ever since she moved in with us five years ago I've found it easier to think of my mother as less than whole.

I wish now that I hadn't equated her jumbled language and physical deterioration with loss of self and awareness. I vow to talk to her as I would anyone else.

On Valentine's Day, Mom enjoys looking at new family photos; she laughs at a picture of Andrew, now age fourteen, and how he's let his straight brown hair grow below his shoulders. I point to a family portrait we took in Ben's parents' living room on Chinese New Year. "There's Ben's younger brother, the one who walked you down the aisle when we got married."

She says something as soft and light as her breath. I hold my own breath as if to hear better, and in the silence the words form in my brain. I did hear her, and I understood. She said, "I have a brother"—tentatively, as if she wasn't quite sure of the fact, or the thought made her feel sad because she missed him. This spark in her, this connection between us, makes me feel happy.

"Yes, you do! Uncle Jack!"

She nods.

I say, "Your brother Jack," and she smiles. Jack is seven years younger than my mother, and in robust good health. He tells me he bikes fifty miles a week and walks four miles a day. He still works part-time remodeling homes, and his mind seems perfectly sharp.

I savor this moment with Mom, then try to continue the conversation.

"We should invite him for another visit, don't you think?"

"Yes." This is firm and clear.

"He hasn't been here in about six months." With this her smile fades into a look of confusion or hurt, so I quickly add, "He lives in Louisiana and it takes him two days to drive here, so he doesn't get up here very often."

Gauging the look on her face—still sad or confused—I try to reassure her some more. "I'll talk to him tonight. I'll invite him back up for a visit. Would you like that?"

She still looks puzzled and doesn't answer. In a split second her pleasure in remembering her brother got pushed out by something else, and I can only guess by what. Maybe I spoke too many sentences in a row for her to follow. Maybe she doesn't understand why I would be the one to call Jack and not her. Maybe she's disappointed that he's not nearby and can't visit immediately. I can't pretend to know. What I can do is accept that it's all okay.

"I was talking to your mom the other day about her dog." It's a new RA, one of three new RA's I don't recognize today. She's stopped at the table in the dining room where I'm showing my mother the photos, which include pictures of Trinka before we had to put her to sleep. For the last few years we took care of Trinka, when she lost her sight and hearing, she stopped barking and nipping and grew gentle. Ben, the kids, and I found ourselves more attached to her.

I had not yet told Mom of Trinka's death. I didn't want her to feel sad. Now I speak to my mother as someone who does not need, and would not want, to be protected from the facts of life and death.

I hold her hand and say, "Unfortunately, Mom, we had to put Trinka down. She was fourteen and really sick."

"Oh!" she says, her eyes wide.

"We had to put her to sleep. She died last fall."

I pause, then say, "She had a tumor in her brain. We had part of the tumor removed from behind her eye, but it didn't help." I try to keep it simple but truthful.

After the initial alarm Mom's face looks blank.

"I brought her here to say good-bye to you, Mom, right before we took her to the vet to have her put to sleep. You petted her on your lap." I was so sad about Trinka's death that I had to ask Ben to take her to be put down (and at the vet's he cried, too).

Mom's eyes look dark. I stop talking, and make room at the table for whatever reaction Mom might experience.

Another day, as I drive Mom to the dentist for a teeth cleaning, I say, "Look at that beautiful old church, Mom. It's such a lovely building, isn't it?" I point to the right, out the passenger-side window, but even though Mom's looking at me, not out the window, I continue. "It's the Presbyterian Church, like the one you used to go to when you were growing up, the one in LeRoy. You got married there."

"Sure!" she says. I take my own eyes off the road long enough to give her a quick smile. I can see through the corner of my eye that she continues to watch my face intently. A block down I point to another church.

"That's the United Methodist Church. I'm thinking of going there."

Softy, but as clear as if we were sitting in the car ten years ago, Mom says, "Why is that?" She sounds surprised.

I feel tingly. We're having a real conversation. Does my mother want to know why I'm considering going to church because she remembers that I've never been a churchgoer? Or does she say those particular three words because it's a simple and polite phrase in response to anyone saying that they want to try something new? Who knows? I'm thrilled to make that connection with her intellect, to talk, once again, with my mother who was always curious about everything in the world, always interested in me.

"I'm thinking of going there because they have a female pastor. They're open-minded. And they're really nice people. Andrew and Morgan went to preschool there." I think about how I want to be more spiritual, and how I might explain that in one or two sentences, but it's time to pull into the driveway of the dentist's house. Mom points up at the large sign on the front porch that's white in the shape of a molar. She laughs.

After the appointment I swing into a fast-food drive-through to get her a chocolate milkshake, an easy treat that doesn't involve getting out of the car. Coaching Mom in and out of the passenger side of my van has become nearly impossible. She no longer seems able to translate my verbal directions—"Scoot your bottom over, Mom," or, "Lift your other leg"—into movement. She stands for long moments clutching the door handle, unwilling or unable to bend, rigid as a plank.

When I pull up at Elm Haven, I have to call on my cell phone for a staff member to run outside and help me persuade Mom to climb out of the car. Inside, Mom offers a huge smile and multiple hugs to the RAs in the living room. She seems to see them as long-lost friends who mean the world to her. I'm happy for her.

Another Search for Home

By February of 2010 Mom has declined so much that she spends most of her time dozing in the small TV room at the end of her hallway, eats little, and ignores the group activities. I no longer see the sense in paying nearly $6,000 a month for a private facility when she qualified for Medicaid months ago. I ramp up my research of local nursing homes, and file a Medicaid application with the county Department of Social Services.

My neighbor, Karen, who led our community discussion of dementia, tells me about the book, *Life Worth Living: How Someone You Love Can Still Enjoy Life in a Nursing Home* by William H. Thomas, M.D. Though I'm skeptical of the title's promise, I find myself intrigued with Thomas's approach to elder care. In 1991, Thomas, a Harvard-educated physician and geriatrician, and his wife, Jude, founded an international, not-for-profit organization called The Eden Alternative®. Its fundamental tenet is that nursing homes must be redesigned, from the physical environment to programs to staffing, to combat what they call the "three plagues" of institutional care: loneliness, helplessness, and boredom.

Thomas envisioned nursing homes that practice The Eden Alternative as more like a garden than a facility—a "human habitat" filled with life—plants, animals, frequent visits by children, and impromptu interactions with the staff. The Eden Alternative also models a new "culture of care." It's part of the staff's job to not only dress and feed the residents but to sit down and talk with them, to give them a hug if they want one. Elders are encouraged to give as well as to receive this kind of affection. They're offered a range of meaningful activities each day. Caring, and the warmth of human contact, are more important than treatment and schedules.

Unfortunately we lack nursing homes in our area that fully embrace all aspects of The Eden Alternative philosophy. Karen knows many Eden Alternative leaders through her work, and recommends an excellent nursing home on The Eden Alternative Registry two hours away, the closest. I call the home and arrange a tour, but in the end decide that I'd rather find a good place within a half hour's drive that allows me to visit my mother more often and be readily available if she has to go to the hospital.

Around this time I also learn from my neighbor Karen about a recent initiative of The Eden Alternative, "Eden at Home." Eden at Home brings the philosophies of The Eden Alternative to care at home, helping to improve the quality of life for elders living at home and those who care for them. As I learn about Eden at Home, I wonder how those months my mother lived with us could have been different for our whole family if Eden at Home had existed at that time.

I learn that care at home can easily fall into a replication of the kind of care found in an institution: care that is task- and schedule-oriented instead of person-directed, with interactions that exhaust, frustrate, and deplete everyone involved. Eden at Home emphasizes not aging in place, but aging in community. According to Dr. Thomas, its founder, Eden at Home "teach[es] people how to go beyond care giving. There's this idea, which is very common in our culture, that care giving is a 'pair' relationship: a caregiver and the person getting cared for. It's a one-on-one relationship and other people help, if they can. And that's actually not the way care has been given in most of human history, when care needs were distributed across a clan or tribe or family network.

"So we try to help people build 'care partner networks,' so that the elder is a part of that care partner network, along with maybe a daughter, and maybe a friend from church."

Would I have felt less overwhelmed when Mom lived with us if I had been familiar with Eden at Home? If there had been a social worker or counselor in our area back then who had been trained as an Eden Associate to work with caregivers (as there are now), I suspect that I would have felt less pressure to be the center of my mother's new life. I might also have learned much earlier to see my mother not simply as another responsibility weighing me down, but as a whole, feeling, complicated individual with her own needs—as Judy.

Karen also tells me about another alternative to traditional nursing homes called The Green House Project. Bill Thomas, co-founder of The Eden Alternative, started The Green House Project in 2003 to encourage the growth of nursing homes built not as large, hospital-like institutions, but as clusters of small houses, each with six to ten residents and a completely revamped culture of care.

Their website explains that the "green" in The Green House model means "growth." "The intentionally designed environment, from the open kitchen to the yard, promotes opportunities for elders to live to their fullest potential. Green House homes are designed to let in the natural world, through plenty of sunlight, plants and garden areas, and outdoor access." To change the culture of elder care, "the Green House model focuses on deinstitutionalizing elders, moving to a small house setting, changing the organizational structure, and providing sustainable skilled nursing care in a truly home like environment and with a philosophy that supports continued growth, engagement, and meaning for elders." Green Houses provide all of the clinical care received at a nursing home, but in a homelike, intimate setting with more interaction and affection between staff and residents, and more flexibility to care for elders—not on a schedule, but according to the elders' needs and preferences. Each elder has their own private bedroom and bathroom, and common areas are designed to resemble a private home, with all bedrooms facing a central living room with a fireplace, a small, open kitchen, and one large dining room table.

According to the blogstream Changing Aging, cofounded by Thomas, "the Green House model enhances the quality of life of an elder by emphasizing privacy, dignity, meaningful activity, relationships, and independence as well as improved quality of care." Instead of working all day in segregated tasks where one staff member does the cooking, another the housekeeping, and another the social interaction with residents in planned activities, all staff members are trained in every area, such as safe food handling, personal care, cooking, planning activities, and light housekeeping, and act as almost-family members caring for someone at home. Staff members feel closer to the residents in a Green House home than in a traditional nursing home, enjoy their work more, and turnover is minimal.

I wonder, though, if a Green House could truly give my mother the level of physical care that she needs in the later stages of dementia. With further research I learn that it could. According to the Green House Project literature online, "seventy-five percent

More About the Green House Project

With the financial support of the Robert Wood Johnson Foundation ($12 million since 2002), a non-profit organization called NCB Capital Impact has coordinated most of the creation and testing of The Green House Project. In the fall of 2011, RWJF will donate another $10 million to help NCB Capital Impact bring The Green House Project to low-income communities, the first part of RWJF's new $100 million "impact capital" campaign to encourage partnerships to fund Green Houses in areas that would not normally attract investors.

By September 2011 there will be 113 Green Houses open in 29 states, with another 227 in development. According to the developer of one Green House project, "Green House® operators report increased occupancy, higher satisfaction levels from residents, family and staff, less decline in 'Activities of Daily Living,' dramatic decrease in staff turnover, reduced incidence of depression, less use of medications, and strong testimonials to improved functionality and overall quality of life by elders' family members. Operating costs are proving to be equivalent to current nursing home costs." Care can be paid for by private insurance, Medicare in a limited number of situations, and, if the home is licensed as a nursing home, by Medicaid. If it's a licensed assisted living facility, Medicaid reimbursement depends on the state's particular assisted living regulations. An average of fifty percent or more of Green House residents are on Medicaid.

The AARP calls the project "a model for aging that supports growth," and Long-Term Living magazine calls it one of the "Top Ten Senior Design Innovations."

of Green House elders have some form of dementia...The Green House model is not just for the healthiest seniors. In fact, the range of limitations found in Green House homes is comparable to what you would see in nursing homes."

I learn that several times a day, nurses visit, taking notes on laptop computers or wireless hand-held devices, and are always on call. In his book *What Are Old People For? How Elders Will Change the World*, Thomas explains that "professional nurses enter into and work within the Green House using the home health care metaphor and thus have no need for a fixed base of operations...The nurses' station, long a fixture of the long-term care institution, has no place in a Green House... The people of the Green House counter the tendency to medicalize their home by asking, 'Can we find this in our neighbors' homes?' If not, then its use in the Green House must be seriously questioned." Doctors, social workers, and physical therapists are on call.

I wish that there had been a Green House open in our area when my mother first needed to leave Greenway. If Mom were living in a Green House licensed as a nursing home, she would have enjoyed long, deep relationships with the staff for all of the last years of her life; she would have received the same services as in an assisted living facility or a nursing home; when needed, Medicaid would have taken over payment; she would never have had to move again; and it would have been a true home. I realize now that a Green House would have been ideal.

Sadly, when researching nursing homes for my mother, I discover that the only Green Houses currently open in New York State are three hours away. (Others, two hours away, will open in 2011.) Deeply disappointed, I seek the best nursing home in our city, preferably one that's familiar with The Eden Alternative, even if they're not officially certified as an Eden Alternative home. Our city has three nursing homes, plus a high-end, private-pay continuing care facility. My first choice is a mostly private-pay nursing home on a shady residential side street. I've heard great things about this facility, and when I visit with the assistant director, I like all the green plants hanging from baskets along the main hallway, and the down-home country motif of the dining room with its gingham curtains and wicker centerpieces. The residents seem happy enough, activities abound, and it's clean. I assume the facility must have at least a few beds set aside for Medicaid patients, and the assistant director suggests that they can take Mom "as soon as a bed becomes available." But even though I assure them that I can pay for her care until her Medicaid application is approved, I never hear back from them. I call and leave messages, then finally give up.

My second choice is Woodside, the nursing home where Mom received physical therapy for her fractured pelvis in 2007. Back then I appreciated the professionalism of the staff, but never liked the facility's sterile, hospital-like atmosphere. Since the third option in town has a poor reputation, Woodside appears to be our only choice. From my prior experience with Woodside, I doubt they follow the recommendations of The Eden Alternative. This worries and saddens me.

Part V

THE NURSING HOME

Four Kinds of Pain

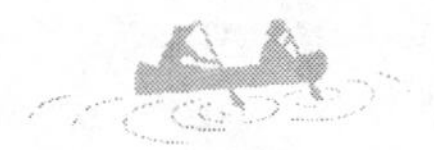

In April 2010, the Elm Haven RAs find Mom on the floor of her bedroom in the middle of the night. She's apparently unhurt, but the next day she's walking hunched over and looks as if she's in pain. I drive her to the E.R., where they tell us that she's lacerated her labia but it will soon heal.

In the E.R., I spoon-feed her for the first time. A nurse has mixed an antibiotic into applesauce, and when I offer Mom one small plastic spoonful after another, we look at each other quizzically, each of us with a half smile. Mom's eyes twinkle at mine. Suspecting that she might feel embarrassed, I say, "I bet you're not used to my feeding you."

As clear as the beep of her blood pressure cuff, Mom says, "I was just thinking that."

I nearly fall off my chair.

The next day when I visit, Mom is just as talkative, though much of what she says is garbled, or so soft I can't hear it. I learn later that when people with dementia take antibiotics, they sometimes experience a temporary period of lucidity. A few researchers believe that Alzheimer's disease is caused by infection, and that antibiotics can briefly halt or reverse the symptoms. No one recommends taking antibiotics all the time, however, and they are not a cure.

Later in April I learn that my mother's application for Medicaid has been denied. Medicaid considers the $100,000 I placed into my mother's checking account to be a "gift." Now they insist that the money be spent down before she'll qualify. That's a lot of money for us to lose.

I warn any family caregiver I meet that if they are paying their parent's bills to never transfer their own money into their parent's checking account; if you support your parent financially, use your own checks. If you sell property that your parent transferred to you before your state's Medicaid look-back period, as Mom did, keep the proceeds of the sale far away from your parents' bank accounts, even if you plan on using all or part of the funds for their care. In all my hours in caregiver support meetings, I never heard about this. I urge my lawyer, who gives presentations to caregiver groups about legal paperwork, to be sure and tell people to beware.

This lawyer will help me file an appeal of this decision, and she will also submit a new application. She tells me we're more likely to win if Mom's already living in a nursing home. It's time to move her. As Mom's health has declined to the point where she might be better off in a nursing home, I agree to try to find her a place within a month, by early May. I cross my fingers that Woodside will have an available bed.

My attorney uses a legal loophole that will allow us to salvage about $30,000 of the $60,000 remaining in my mother's checkbook. Out of that $30,000 we must pay the attorney fee of $5,000.

• • •

When I think of the bare, white halls of Woodside where Mom did rehab, I want to fill it with smiles and hugs, touch and laughter. Maybe one or two of her favorite RAs from Elm Haven would agree to visit her each week for pay. I want Mom to have that continuity; I don't want her to lose all her friends from Elm Haven as she did when we moved her there from Greenway. Zeisel's book *I'm Still Here* has convinced me that Mom remains capable of building new relationships, and that she might feel hurt if she never saw the Elm Haven staff again. As I can't visit her all the time, I want Mom to have as many "angels who fall from heaven" in her life as possible. I ask Diane, the director at Elm Haven, to pass on my request to the RAs.

Only one RA—Gina—expresses interest, but she tells me on the phone that she loves my mother and that she would be happy to continue to see her. Her own mother, she says, lived at Woodside and passed away there five years ago. I will end up hiring her to see Mom for an hour two days a week, and she sends me lovely updates by email. "Have you ever had one of those days," she writes, "and something someone says or does makes it better? I had one of those days with your mom today. She was all smiles and laughs, and someone said they hadn't seen her smile and laugh that way in a while. It just made me feel good!"

Another angel, Carol, a neighbor who's a massage therapist, specializes in bodywork for elders. I hire her to offer my mother a weekly hand massage. Soon Mom lets Carol massage her shoulders, arms, and lower legs while they listen to music. Carol reads out loud, or talks, and holds Mom's hand.

I'm grateful to each of these women. One of the saddest parts of my mother's dementia has been the loss of frequent contact with her old friends. These women are new friends, and good ones.

Rebound

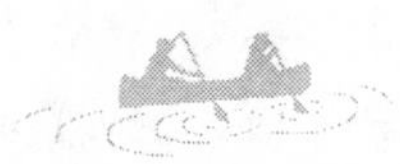

On May 1, 2010, Ben and I move my mother from memory care at Elm Haven to the secure dementia floor at Woodside Nursing Home. It maddens me that the reason I must move her, for the sixth time in five years, is a quirk of public policy: Medicaid in our state will pay for nursing home care, but not for someone to spoon-feed her at a memory care place like Elm Haven.

In Barbara Ehrenreich's book *Bright-Sided: How the Relentless Promotion of Positive Thinking Has Undermined America*, she argues that when individuals in crisis feel pressure to make the best of a horrible situation, they are, in effect, letting the rest of society off the hook. If we take pride in struggling as rugged individuals, we expect—and get—less support from society as a whole.

"To be disappointed, resentful, or downcast," Ehrenreich says, "is to be a 'victim' and a 'whiner.'" Arlene, the woman with the red lipstick from my support group, says that, as caregivers, "we are not victims." I believe she means that we can choose to be proactive for our loved ones, to demand what our loved ones would want if they could speak for themselves. She also means that we can choose to take care of our own well-being, to not act as martyrs. But I believe that people living with dementia, and their family caregivers, *are* often victims, plain and simple—not because of timidity or passivity, but because of shortsighted public policy. So much could be done, so easily, using just common sense.

I have filed the appeal with Medicaid, and am waiting for a hearing to be scheduled. Until I win the appeal, or Medicaid accepts the new application submitted by my attorney, we must pay for Mom's care, at $230 a day. I know that in New York State Medicaid will pay for nursing home care retroactively for three months, if income and assets are within the required limits. I assume that we will be reimbursed eventually for Woodside's charges.

Before we leave Elm Haven I ask the staff to pose for a photo with Mom. She's seemed happier during these two and a half years with them than I've seen her in fifteen years. Taking her away from them makes today one of the saddest days of my life.

The morning of Mom's move, I go to Woodside by myself to decorate her corner of her double room; that way, she'll see her familiar things when she arrives. When I step off the elevator, the common room looks quite different from when Mom did rehab there three years earlier. The old nursing station, an imposing desk built into the floor at the back of the common room, has been removed and replaced with a small medication cart on wheels. The white cinder block walls have been painted light green, a wallpaper border of green leaves and flowers runs along the walls, and the old white tile floor has been replaced with light-brown vinyl flooring that looks like wood. There are new comfortable chairs and couches, ivory curtains on the large windows overlooking the courtyard, and lots of plants. Where once there was a large flat-screen TV on a wall, one that was almost always on, there is now a small TV that

I will discover is only on if they're playing an old movie. Usually they play music on the CD player.

I will learn that Woodside has a new director, a young woman who started her career as a recreation therapist, and also many new staff. The physical therapist, nurses, and social workers I remember from Mom's rehab are gone. I find the new nurses to be much friendlier, and several young recreation aides sprinkle their bubbly enthusiasm and affection around the common room like cinnamon sugar on toast.

Mom's roommate is a lovely woman named Elaine, about Mom's age, with moist, friendly eyes. Elaine shows some signs of confusion but can still speak clearly, feed herself, and walk on her own without a walker. I would think she'd do well in a memory care place such as Elm Haven, and I wonder how she ended up at Woodside. Perhaps, like Mom, she's run out of savings, or perhaps her family knew of no other alternative. Nearly every time I visit, I see her sitting in the common room, placid, her eyes down and her hands folded in her lap. When I greet her she immediately sparks to life. I feel grateful each time I see Elaine that Mom has such a sweet, "with it" roommate.

Mom will sleep in the bed away from the window, and a nurse helps me move the bed against the wall and crank it lower to the floor, so Mom will be less likely to hurt herself if she rolls out of bed. At night, the aides will tuck a body pillow along the length of the bed, attach Mom's nightgown to an alarm, and, now that Mom's less likely to try to get up on her own, they place a thick rubber mat on the floor next to the bed.

A young man from the maintenance department secures the large framed painting from the cottage of the two white sailboats on a deep blue lake onto the wall over Mom's bed. I hang the framed photo of her in her canoe, the blown-up portrait of me at eighteen, and others: Mom when she was younger, her parents, my brother, and Andrew and Morgan. I label the photos ("I canoed 30 miles around Silver Lake with my miniature Schnauzer Khara Mia," "Mom and Dad," and "This is me") in case Mom can still read them and the staff are willing to talk to her about these images from her past. Right behind her bed, I hang the soft, fabric Christmas wreath with a partridge and pears that a friend made for her thirty years ago. I plug in a small lamp on the end table; that way she can have some soft light instead of only the harsh light of the fluorescent tube on the wall behind her bed. As Mom's storage space is much less generous here than at Elm Haven, with a closet one and a half feet wide and five small drawers, I winnow her clothes down to the most essential. I label the drawers to help the staff find each item in a hurry. Outside their shared bathroom, up high near the ceiling, hangs a solid metal rack meant to hold a television. I don't want Mom to lie in bed staring at a TV, or the ugly, empty rack; I place a large pot of artificial red geraniums up there and the maintenance guy secures it with a thin, cabled chain.

Over the next few weeks the staff will often comment on how much they love the decorations and pictures. Though I've created a familiar nest for Mom in this angular, transitory space, I suspect she's not fooled. Does she know this is a nursing home—her final stop? I worry that beneath her silence she will feel sad or angry.

Indeed, when we move her in later that day, Mom doesn't seem to notice her familiar belongings. Her affect is blank. When we slip out, a nurse sits with Mom on the edge of her bed and puts her arm around her.

In the first six weeks at Woodside Mom eats almost nothing. She continues to forget how to use a fork or spoon, and turns her head away when the aides try to feed her. I make sure they offer her one food at a time, protein first, with only one utensil, and that they offer her at each meal a finger food such as a peanut butter and jelly sandwich.

Nothing helps Mom at this point. She chews on pieces of her paper napkins until I ask the staff to stop giving them to her. Week after week, she loses weight. The head nurse on Mom's floor, a calm and professional woman, tries to reassure me. Many new residents go through a difficult period of adjustment, she says. When she advises me to "give it some time," I try not to worry, but I can't.

One day while I wait by the elevator, a staff member who's waiting with me asks me a question, as if in passing, that I did not anticipate.

"If your mom continues to lose weight, how would you feel about a feeding tube?"

A feeding tube? Is that where they're headed already? I say, "I wouldn't want her to have one. And I know for sure that she wouldn't want one."

A tiny smile flicks across his face but he says nothing more. I wonder why he thinks it's okay to so casually ask me this question, while the head nurse has not.

His question tears me apart. If Mom stops eating and doesn't have a feeding tube inserted into her stomach, she'll starve to death. I research feeding tubes online and see that the tubes can be painful, and if someone like Mom, who forgets why it's there, tugs at it, the hole can get infected. I don't know who to talk to who has experience with these kinds of decisions. I don't yet trust the nursing home staff to do what's best for my mother rather than what their state regulators might want them to do.

I call Dan at the Office for the Aging, who suggests that I call our regional Alzheimer's Association. One of their counselors tells me that the subject of feeding tubes comes up very frequently with caregivers who have a family member with late-stage dementia. I feel tremendous relief just knowing I'm not alone. But when they recommend that I ask our local hospice to visit and evaluate my mother, I waver. This most recent decline has come on so suddenly I'm not ready to think about my mother needing hospice. I talk to some of my neighbors who've had experience with hospice, but I end up not calling.

By mid-June, Mom rebounds. She eats well, even better than she did her last months at Elm Haven. And when the staff members say hello to her, she stretches her arm out towards them, wiggles her fingers, and gives them her signature smile.

It saddens me to think that Mom had such a difficult time at first, but her decline ceases, she seems content, and once again, I can breathe.

The same month, I have my first hearing with a judge from the state Medicaid office to contest their rejection of Mom's application, and it's a debacle. The judge, a large man with a booming voice whose face grows redder each minute, demands that before I can represent my mother, I must produce a letter from her doctor stating that because of her dementia she is unable to attend or understand the hearing. He says my Durable Power of Attorney and Health Care Proxy are insufficient. I get the distinct impression that he'd like nothing better than for her case to go away. I had read the Medicaid application material thoroughly and nowhere did it say that such a letter was necessary for a family member to represent an applicant. The judge rises, grabs his thick folder and storms out.

The county Medicaid officer, a woman who processed the paperwork and sat beside the judge, walks me to the waiting room. "I'm so sorry," she says, flustered. "That's never happened before. I don't know why he did that."

In early July, we are offered a new hearing. I filed a formal request for a different judge, but my request is ignored and we're assigned the same judge. Ben accompanies me as a witness to corroborate my story that the money we put into Mom's account was ours and not meant as a gift to her. We bring a letter from Mom's doctor stating that my mother "has progressive dementia, and to a medical degree of certainty cannot comprehend a Medicaid or any similar hearing." The judge has cooled down; he shows no sign of agitation until he tries to get me to say that the money was a gift: "So you deposited that sum of money into your mother's account to be able to continue to pay her bills. Was that not a gift? How can that not be considered a gift?" He stretches his thick arms out to his side as if to emphasize his point, puffing out his barrel chest like an angry goose. Despite his bluster, I feel hopeful, and half expect that we will win.

By mid-July, though, Medicaid informs me that our appeal has been denied. Fortunately, the second application by the attorney has been approved. My mother now has only the allowed amount of $13,800 in her checking account, and the remaining balance of the $100,000, about $50,000, sits in a different bank account under my name. I must continue to use those funds to pay for her care during a "penalty" period of a number of months equivalent to the amount she was "gifted" divided by the average cost of nursing home care in our area. Since we've been paying for her nursing home care since May, we will need to continue to pay for her care for four more months, through October. We will not receive the retroactive reimbursement we were hoping to get.

In August for my mother's seventy-eighth birthday, I plan a small gathering at Woodside to celebrate her life. On the invitations, I write, "Though she's living with advanced dementia, Mom will delight in your presence. Years ago she wanted a celebration of her life after she passed, but we're sharing our love and affection for her now while she can enjoy it." I suspect that by the following year she might be much less responsive. Now is the time.

Her brother visited a few weeks before, and he doesn't drive up again, but my step-grandmother, the one who took us in when my mother divorced my stepfather, comes, though I'm not sure Mom recognizes her. Bill and Susan, Mom's neighbors from the lake, join us, and Andy, my neighbor who helped Mom visit assisted living places five years ago. I wanted to invite Mom's oldest friends, those from her teaching jobs she kept in touch with, but I can't find her little address book and they're not online. Some of her newest friends attend—Gina the RA from Elm Haven, and Carol, the massage therapist. I sent an invitation to the directors of both Greenway and Elm Haven to invite any staff who might like to see Mom, but only one person aside from Gina arrives—a dining room worker from Greenway who particularly enjoyed my mother. He brings his wife, and it feels lovely to think that someone at Greenway remembers her fondly.

Ben and I cook the meal. I bake Mom's angel food cake—the kind she used to make for my birthday—and we invite all of the staff at Woodside to join us. I display photos of my mother and her family, and throughout the party, a harpist plays "Clair de Lune" and other of my mother's favorite pieces. It's a small, serene party, and though she says little, Mom holds people's hands, smiles, and locks onto their eyes with hers. She listens closely and laughs right on cue. I'm not sure which guests she recognizes and remembers, but that's okay.

Small Pleasures

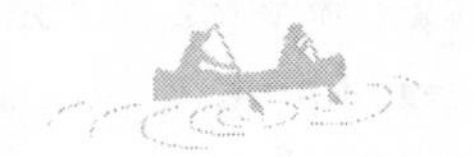

In September, I attend an all-day gerontology conference at a local college, eager to learn the latest insights into dementia care. Dr. G. Allen Power, author of the book *Dementia Beyond Drugs: Changing the Culture of Care*, describes to the audience the traditional view of dementia as tragic, irreversible, costly, and burdensome for caregivers and society. Certainly that's how I used to think of dementia. But dementia merely represents a shift, he says, in someone's perception of the world. People with dementia can still learn new things, and there continues to be the potential for growth and enjoyment of life.

I've seen this potential in Mom's transition to Woodside. She seems to recognize the staff as they walk toward her even before they see her or talk to her. She's ready to smile at them even before they give her a big "Hello, Judy!" In the same way, she seems to recognize the man who volunteers to lead their sing-along time, and she's developed a relationship not only with Gina, the RA from Elm Haven she's known for three years, but also with Carol, the massage therapist who's known her for only a few months.

During the five months my mother has lived at Woodside I have avoided visiting her more often than every week or two because I've felt like our visits are a bit superficial and forced, plastic, as if we do not really understand each other. But in our last few visits I've felt her joy in simple things—the deep blue, cloudless sky above the courtyard, and watching my new miniature Schnauzer puppy, Shadow, bounce around like a rabbit. She seems to cherish eating a brownie, and touching my face. She listens to me carefully.

"Do you feel cold?" I ask her on a brisk fall day as we sit in the sun in the courtyard by the crispy, brown stalks of summer flowers.

"No."

"Would you like some more brownie?"

"Yes!"

"Mom, Andrew turned fifteen last week. Can you believe he's fifteen already?" Her eyes grow wide.

If I pay attention, I see that her responses are all spot-on. Judy is still "here." But for how long?

When my mother moved into Woodside, she still walked with a walker, but so slowly that the staff used a wheelchair to get her to activities and meals in a timely manner. For a few months they tried to walk with her as much as possible, but now she sits all day in a facility-issued black wheelchair. I am still uncertain whether she was doomed to lose her ability to walk at this particular time, or whether it happened because a wheelchair is more expedient for the staff.

I understand the desire for expedience. Her mobility issues have made me reluctant to try to take her out into the world. I did try to find a van service I could pay to pick her up in her wheelchair and take her to my house or a concert. The local ambulance company offers a wheelchair service for non-emergencies, but it's $80 each way. I know of no other alternative.

Her incontinence complicates matters. She needs to have her Depends changed every few hours. I don't want her to feel uncomfortable, away too long from the aides who whisk her so efficiently in and out of the bathroom.

In any case, she now takes only a few steps from wheelchair to bed or toilet, and walks with a walker only a few times a week for physical therapy. When I want to take her for a walk in the wheelchair, and I try to lift her feet onto her foot rests, her legs are so rigid I can barely move them.

I find, in a pile of Mom's old letters, the tiny address book for which I'd been searching. I telephone Mom's first 12-step sponsor from thirty years ago to see if she'd like to visit. When Mom sees this woman, she shakes with excitement, trembling as I've never seen her before. Though it's probably been twenty years since they saw each other, I'm certain she remembers her. The woman lives two hours away but promises to visit again, and to bring a fiddle so she can play some music.

On her way out, the woman says to me, "Take care of *you*," just like Mom used to do.

Two weeks later another old friend of my mother's, a younger woman who used to teach Mom aerobics twenty-five years ago, comes to visit, and again Mom vibrates with what looks very much like recognition and joy.

In October, Medicaid takes over paying for most of Mom's care. I write a check from her account each month to the nursing home for an amount equivalent to her Social Security and pension income. Medicaid now pays for her Depends, her Medicare premium, and her prescriptions. Every six months or so, I give Woodside a check for her personal account, to pay for her haircuts. Medicaid allows her to keep only $50 a month in income.

My attorney advises that Mom keep her Blue Cross and Blue Shield supplemental insurance, as it may give her coverage that she wouldn't have otherwise; some providers, for example, do not accept Medicaid, and private insurance may cover a medication or procedure that Medicaid does not. If I were to cancel her supplemental insurance, Medicaid would simply require that the money go to the nursing home.

Mom has few expenses, and her monthly bank balance will hover around $6,000.

I'm relieved that she's been taken under the wing of the state, but thankful she knows nothing of her impoverishment.

It's December, and the winter solstice is celebrated again in our community. I want my mother to be able to join me as she has for the past five years, but I'm still puzzled by how to get her around. It finally occurs to me to call our city's bus service for the elderly and disabled. I assume that they won't have service on a Saturday evening, and I'm right, but they tell me that I can file an application for my mother to qualify for transportation guaranteed by the Americans with Disabilities Act. A special bus with a wheelchair lift can take her almost anywhere around the city, evenings and weekends included, for just a few dollars each way. I'm thrilled, and so grateful.

Amae

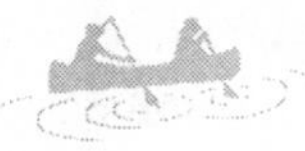

I find the old report of my mother's neuropsychological exam from 1997 and read it again carefully in case I missed something. The exam found only a slight cognitive decline at that time—mostly just her obsessive-compulsive attention to detail—but two words jump out at me that I don't remember seeing before: "bipolar disorder."

Apparently the psychiatrist who ordered the exam had already determined this diagnosis. The "hypomania" referred to in the report—her rapid, excessive speech—is typical of bipolar II disorder, a less severe form of bipolar disorder in which the patient does not experience a full-blown manic episode. Why had I never noticed these words? I wonder. I probably found it too difficult to confront the possibility that, like my father and brother, my mother also had a major mental illness.

This time I force myself to stop and stare at the words, to let them sink in.

Bipolar II disorder would explain much of the strange, antisocial behavior and irritability that first concerned me sixteen years ago, around the time Mom kicked Ben and me out of the cottage when I was six months pregnant.

I learn that bipolar II disorder is often misdiagnosed as major depression because patients usually seek help when they are in a depressed, not in a manic, state. What I saw in my mother at that time did lean more to depression—sleeping odd hours, withdrawal from friends, letting the house go. The manic side might have been, in addition to her rapid and excessive speech, how she often could not sleep at all because she felt excited about something, such as an upcoming visit with me. I see from the report that Mom was taking lithium, a common treatment for bipolar disorder.

I write a letter to Mom's old psychiatrist to ask if she could tell me why she diagnosed my mother with bipolar II disorder. It would explain a lot of my mother's behavior, I write, but it's also important for me to know as the mother of two teenagers who already carry the genetic burden of their grandfather's and uncle's mental illness.

I mail a similar letter to Dr. Galvin, Mom's old primary doctor.

I hope to hear from at least one of them, as I don't know whom else to ask.

I may never fully understand my mother's history and diagnoses, and I may have to live with some uncertainty, but it gnaws at me. I wish someone could hand me a definitive diagnosis. It would go a long way not just toward forgiveness—that I've reached—but toward peace of mind as I age myself, if I could know what to look for in my own aging brain. As the only person in my immediate family of origin who is not mentally ill, I am fearful.

• • •

Today, I want fresh air for Mom, sunshine on her face as she rides the wheelchair lift into the bus, the view through the windows of the snow-covered trees embroidered in white, the gentle bounce of the tires over the rutted streets. We're headed to a college cinema for a screening of the movie *Mary Poppins*. Audience members will dress up in character, and the lyrics to the songs will be typed on the screen to help people sing along.

We wait in the lobby by the fish tank for the wheelchair bus to arrive. I tell Mom that Morgan had a sleepover the night before and that the girls kept me awake until one o'clock, then woke me at seven o'clock. Mom tilts her head to the side and shakes her head almost imperceptibly, like "tsk, tsk," her eyes wide and locked on mine. I love talking to my mother now because I realize that she understands almost everything I'm saying. Today, though, I think not about our time together in this present moment, but about the years past when we fought and I would never have dreamed of feeling so tender toward her.

Yesterday I found an old journal in which I'd written about that summer evening in 1995 shortly after Ben and I were married when Mom kicked us out. "You remember that day," I said to Ben. He nodded and grimaced. I said, "You must have wondered what the heck you got yourself into."

"I did. But it was too late!"

How, I wonder now in the lobby, can I look lovingly at a woman who once treated me, and my new husband, so monstrously? Is it just that she's unable to pick a fight, that she's defanged? Have I forgotten her bizarre behavior? No, I remember. But it's past, and I can see reasons why she did all that she did, whether from depression or anxiety, obsessive-compulsive personality disorder, bipolar II disorder, or early dementia. The forgiveness I feel comes not from complete understanding, but from acknowledging that I most likely will never find an explanation for all of her behavior.

Today Mom looks as gentle as a new mother. I feel as if we are reunited in what the Japanese call "amae" (pronounced "a-mah-yeh"), the protective, dependent cocoon of mother and child. Some say that in Japanese culture adults often wish to return to this overindulgent kind of mothering in their relationships to their parents, teachers and bosses, to the state of always feeling accepted and forgiven. Through dementia, Mom and I have returned to that state. We've flown back through the years to my first months in her arms as an infant, to those precious hours in the afternoons after her teaching job, when we snuggled together in our living room in the white wicker rocking chair. In our hearts, we are each safe and forgiven.

But, of course, not all visits are peaceful. One day, as we sit at the end of her hallway next to a large window, I ask Mom if she'd like to give my puppy a dog treat. She nods, and I hand her the small brown nugget. Immediately she pops it into her mouth. I should have known better, I think to myself. "Mom, spit it out, okay?" Puzzlement flashes through her eyes and she furrows her brow but she keeps chewing. Finally she opens her mouth but the dog treat is gone, dissolved on her tongue. The wave of guilt I feel swirls with a sharp pang of sadness.

Later in the same visit I offer her a cup of ginger ale in one of the small plastic cups the nurses give residents to use for water to take their medication. Mom has been sucking on the bottom corner of her pink sweater, sucking, sucking, as if trying to get liquid out of it. She can still drink from a cup, or from a straw, with prompting, though often she seems confused about what to do with the cup after she drinks.

"Let me help you, Mom. Let me help you get your sweater out of your mouth so you can drink some ginger ale."

Mom shakes her head, and squeezes the cup, buckling its sides. I try to take it.

"Mom, let go. I don't want this to spill all over you and all over me."

She glares at me and yanks the cup away. The ginger ale spills into a circle on her lap.

"Great," I say. "Nice going, Mom." I know as soon as I say it that I shouldn't have, that Mom doesn't deserve this flash of venom. But there it is.

Mom deflates, as if ashamed that she's made a mess, and hurt by my words. She lets me take the cup and she drops the sweater from her mouth. She stares at her lap while I find an aide to change her pants.

I end this visit by sitting with my mother and her roommate Elaine in the common room, talking to Elaine while she pets my puppy on her lap. I'm pleased that Mom seems to enjoy listening to us chat and watching the dog, but I also feel relieved to take a break from paying such close attention to my mother.

My visits with Mom over the past few years have taught me many lessons I carry into the rest of my life. The foremost is that I can slow down throughout the day and be more aware of what I'm thinking, how I feel, and how I react toward others. I've started classes in meditation called "Mindfulness-Based Stress Reduction." I have worked with a life coach to question my thoughts and the assumptions I make about myself and others.

I tend to judge both myself and other people harshly, and I assume that others will judge me harshly in return. (When Mom was in her 12-step program she admitted doing the same thing, and called it "stinkin' thinkin'.") Even though I lose my cool with

Mom once in a great while, as I did the day I said "Nice going, Mom," for the most part visiting her has taught me how to slow down and think before I react. This has been especially helpful with my teenagers—to listen to them and be fully "present."

I am also much more appreciative now of my husband's personality. I knew he was generous, of course, but I used to think that he was too passive, too flexible for his own good. I realize now that he simply didn't grow up with all of the drama that I did, that he's comfortable with himself in any situation and not easily thrown off balance. He gives me a feeling of safety and acceptance that I'd never known before. His example teaches me how to let go of my guilt, worry, and judgments. In 2011 I will face these painful habits head-on by returning to my own 12-step meetings for adult children of alcoholics.

The immediacy of life with dementia has brought me the gift of awareness—awareness not only of my many imperfections, but of my completeness. Like my mother, I am flawed but whole, challenged but resilient.

Is It Alzheimer's, or Not?

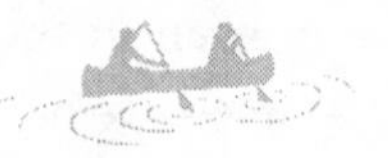

In March of 2011 I read for the first time about a kind of dementia called Frontotemporal Dementia. According to the collection of essays in the book *What If It's Not Alzheimer's?: A Caregiver's Guide to Dementia*, edited by Lisa and Gary Radin, Frontotemporal Dementia, or FTD, is the most common dementia after Alzheimer's disease in people under age sixty-five, and usually develops between the ages of forty and seventy. FTD affects the brain's frontal and temporal lobes, which control behavior, personality, and language. People with FTD typically act inappropriately, insensitively, and with poor judgment, and can also seem apathetic. They struggle to speak clearly and have difficulty understanding instructions. Eventually they lose their speech and comprehension entirely.

I wonder if Mom has FTD. Her early difficulty with language began with struggles with spelling. As a retired teacher she found her inability to spell words she always knew as particularly dismaying. She started to type letters to me on her computer—the word processor being the only function she could operate—in order to use spell check.

I learn that early-stage FTD is often misdiagnosed as Alzheimer's disease, as a personality disorder, or as a psychological condition, "only to later find out," as the Radins write in their introduction, that "there is a neurodegenerative condition that is the cause of the matter." Indeed, when Mom's old psychiatrist writes me back, she admits that while she strongly suspected bipolar disorder, she does not know enough about Frontotemporal Dementia to consider that diagnosis. (Dr. Gavin never responded to my letter.)

I suspect FTD because what first concerned me about my mother's behavior years ago was not the memory loss typical of Alzheimer's disease, but episodes of poor judgment, antisocial behavior, and lack of empathy. That summer day in 1995, when she kicked us out, is a prime example. In her mid-sixties, Mom alienated not only me, but many of her long-time friends, who found her stubborn and insensitive. An old 12-step friend ended their friendship after Mom visited her and refused to stop smoking in her house. Another friend of many years stopped visiting because of Mom's compulsion to talk non-stop about the importance of investing in mutual funds.

In one of the essays in *What If It's Not Alzheimer's?*, Murray Grossman calls this kind of behavior in FTD "a disorder of social comportment, particularly a rigid and cold personality with obsessive clinical features." Mom could show that flat affect, lack of compassion, poor judgment, and obsession with discussing topics of little interest to her listeners. Grossman says that this early period of FTD can be a "prolonged period of subtle but insidious change."

Another symptom of FTD is overeating, particularly a craving for sweet food. Mom also now exhibits the "hyper oral" habits of

FTD—mouthing and chewing on objects that are not food, such as napkins and clothing.

As Katherine P. Rankin points out in an essay in *What If It's Not Alzheimer's?*, people with FTD often seem unaware of their difficulties. "Some patients actually become much more easygoing, pleasant, and even more friendly than they were before the onset of their disease." Most of the time, this behavior also characterizes Mom.

On the other hand, when I read Rachel Hadas' book *Strange Relation: A Memoir of Marriage, Dementia, and Poetry*, about her husband who had FTD, much of how she describes her husband does *not* sound like Mom: he became "an increasingly ghost-like non-presence," and, "He is so barely present here and now." Mom is not a ghost; she is still here. She has not lost her comprehension of language, nor her ability to communicate in her own way.

As I write this, brain researchers have developed new tests to distinguish in autopsy the beta amyloid plaques of Alzheimer's disease from the "tau" tangles of FTD. I wish I could know for certain if my mother has FTD, but it will remain a mystery.

Later in April, Mom's brother Jack visits from Louisiana and Ben and I take him out to dinner. I talk about what I've learned about her possible bipolar disorder and frontotemporal dementia. He tells me that when she flew down to Louisiana to visit him and his wife in 1997, Mom's speech was rapid and excessive, just as I remember, and, as she did with me, she talked on and on to him about investing.

She told Jack her psychiatrist was trying to find the right medication for her. She asked Jack, "Do I sound okay to you? Do you think I'm doing all right now, or not?"

"Definitely not," he'd said.

"If I were prone to headaches," he tells me now, "I definitely would have gotten one." He says that while at first she seemed wired and happy, she soon crashed, retreated into the guest bedroom, and refused to come out, just as she would during our visits and when she lived with me.

Dancing Eyes

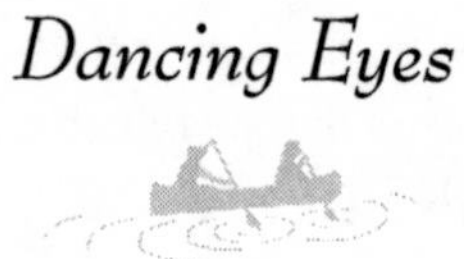

By mid-summer 2011 I tell Ben that we'll have to plan another "life celebration" this year for Mom's seventy-ninth birthday. In some ways she's doing as well as when she first moved into Woodside a year ago, if not better. She does need to be entirely spoon-fed now, as she's forgotten how to maneuver a utensil, but in her care plan meetings the nurses tell me she's eating ninety percent of her food, and her weight is stable. Other than the spoon-feeding, and the need for a wheelchair, she shows no sign of further decline. In this first year at Woodside she's had to go to the E.R. only once, for mild dehydration. She's more engaged with the rich variety of activities here than she was in her last year at Elm Haven—even if she's just listening. If someone cracks a joke across the room, she knows it, and laughs.

When she moved to Woodside, Mom got a new primary care doctor, one of the two doctors who visit the facility. I know now that she could have kept Dr. Claiborne as her doctor (if Dr. Claiborne accepts Medicaid patients). At the time of the move I was thinking only about how much easier it would be for Mom to see a doctor without having to leave the nursing home. Fortunately, her new doctor seems friendly and conscientious. When she's in the hospital for the dehydration, he swings by on rounds and introduces himself to me. Remarking on her smile, he says, "That's not a bad way to be." I tell him that I agree.

I learn later from the nurses that the doctor has taken Mom off of the depression medication she's been on for years. As her health care proxy, I wonder why no one consulted me. The next time I see the doctor, I question him, and he says, "She seems fine without it." Again, he's right; it's hard to distinguish depression from late-stage Alzheimer's. But I sense that, at this point, Mom's medical decisions may be at least partially out of my hands. The nursing home is accountable to Medicaid, not to Mom, or me. I vow, nevertheless, to insist at the next care plan meeting that I be kept informed.

By late 2011, I think of my mother's future and I despair. I imagine my Sunday afternoon visits with Mom in Stage Seven continuing on and on for years, each visit the same as the last. When Sunday rolls around, I would often prefer to stay home with my family. How long will this final stage last? When will she lose that fabulous smile, then the ability to sit without support, hold up her head, chew and swallow? How long will it be before she lies in bed, curled up in a fetal position, rigid, and unseeing? Will she pass away this year, or five years from now?

Despite the moments she enjoys each day, I wonder if my mother has reached the point where she'd prefer to die. I search her eyes for some sign that she's had enough, but all I see are sparks of pleasure and recognition amid sleepiness, bewilderment, and occasional annoyance. If she could speak more than single words, would she say "I love you, but it's time to go"?

I can do nothing but keep watch over her. If she ever needs to go to the E.R., I will make sure that she receives no heroic treatment or invasive procedures. I can help her die in her nursing home bed with hospice care. I hope that Mom will die in her sleep (which, unfortunately, is highly unlikely, statistically), or that she will pass fairly quickly from a massive stroke or pneumonia.

Before each visit, I cringe at the thought of her in this holding pattern—not getting worse, but so far away from how she once was. I despair, that is, until I arrive and sit next to her.

In October I bring her a sweet treat as always, this time a piece of raspberry cheesecake. (Despite what I now know about sugar, insulin resistance, and Alzheimer's, I can't bring myself to cut her off from sugar; any damage it might have done to her neurons is beyond repair, and her immediate pleasure remains most important to me.) I bring the dog, too, and wheel Mom to the family room where the two of us sit and hold hands while Shadow sniffs the floor. I rattle on about what Andrew and Morgan have been up to.

"I'm talking a lot, aren't I, Mom? I'm talking on and on and on. Do you mind that I'm talking so much?" She shakes her head an inch from side to side.

"Remember years ago when you used to talk so much I said it hurt my head?" I smile and look into her eyes; her eyes never leave mine and she gives me a slight nod.

"I'm sorry I hurt your feelings back then. You know, sometimes I wish that we were still sitting at my kitchen table like we did when you lived with me. Sometimes I wish you could talk like that again." I pause and squeeze her hand. "But it's all right, isn't it, Mom? I can still talk with you and I can still understand you even if you have trouble getting the words out. Right?"

She smiles and nods her head almost imperceptibly.

"You might not be able to say much, but I know you're in there. You're right here, aren't you, Mom?" I lean my face closer to hers and she gives me a big smile.

"I love you," I say. I laugh a little and say, "I guess I show my love for you by giving you cheesecake." She tips her chin up and puffs a laugh through her nose that sounds like a tiny set of bellows.

Then I sit back and let silence descend.

After a few moments I say, "You used to make the best birthday cake for me." Her brow crinkles and she shakes her head just the tiniest bit.

"It was angel food cake with pink frosting—fluffy frosting that tasted like marshmallow." Her brow relaxes and her eyes light up.

"I made the same kind of cake for you for your birthday last year." Her eyebrows fly up and her eyes widen.

"Yes, we had the party right here in this room. Bill and Susan came, and a bunch of other people. It was a really nice party. But my cake wasn't as good as yours. The sugar in the frosting came out crunchy. But it tasted good." She smiles.

I always see a reaction if I look closely enough. If she tries to say more than "yes" or "no," I try to repeat what I've heard her say. If it doesn't make much sense and sounds funny, we both laugh.

When I lean down over Mom's wheelchair to say good-bye, I place my arm around her shoulder, my other hand in hers. Her blue eyes are locked on mine, dancing.

I want to tell her how much I love her and appreciate her, but I don't know what words to use. I say, "You're very special, Mom."

Immediately she leans in closer and says "Spe-cial!" Her voice is so crisp, the syllables so clear, I catch my breath. She grins at me as if we're sharing a secret joke.

"Yes, you're very special, Mom. I love you." I wrap her delicate shoulders in a hug, in the softness of my body, and she rests her cheek against mine.

Afterword

As I look back over these seven years, I think of the saying "you know what you know when you know it." Like all caregivers, I did the best I could with the information and support I could find, but I know now that I would do a number of things differently if I had to do it all again.

For one, I was much too trusting of Mom's small town doctor and then her new primary doctor in our city. When Mom lived at the cottage, as soon as she started hoarding and not cleaning and cooking, I wish I had paid more attention and hired a geriatric care manager to visit her. A geriatric care manager could have assessed her ability to care for herself and to drive, and offered us suggestions for the next steps to take. Surely I would not have been able to deny my mother's dementia as long as I did.

I would have found a top-notch neurologist who specializes in dementia and tried to convince my mother to have another neuropsychological exam such as the one she had in 1997. I'd make sure that Mom was tested for conditions that mimic Alzheimer's disease but are reversible, such as vitamin deficiencies and depression. For the neuropsychological assessment, I'd ask the geriatric care manager to help us accurately answer the medical questions. Indeed, I'd follow the advice of Nataly Rubinstein, a geriatric care manager and author of the book *Alzheimer's Disease and Other Dementias: The Caregiver's Complete Survival Guide,* and have the geriatric care manager walk us through each step of the process of receiving an accurate diagnosis.

I would not have believed Mom's primary care doctor when she told me that the available Alzheimer's medications did no good.

I would have done my own research, and convinced the neurologist to at least try these medications to slow the progression of my mother's symptoms. The longer Mom could dress herself, use the bathroom, and feed herself, for example, the longer she could have stayed out of a nursing home.

I would not have rushed into moving Mom into my house. I may have paid for aides to help my mother at the cottage, or convinced my mother to move directly to assisted living, or questioned why I felt confident caring for Mom in my own home, given our history. Though I received credible advice from other caregivers in my support group, my city's Family and Children's Services caregiver counselors, a social worker, an elder care psychologist, and various staff members at her facilities, none of the advice I patched together could have equaled in breadth and depth what I would have learned from an experienced geriatric care manager familiar with all aspects of my mother's life.

On the financial side, I would have paid for the initial geriatric care assessments myself when Mom lived at the cottage. Then, when I handled her finances, I would have swallowed my fear of depleting her savings; the cost of hiring a geriatric care manager would no doubt have saved us some of the money we paid for her facilities—and the cost to our sanity and well-being.

In this alternative universe, if my mother did move into a traditional assisted living facility such as Greenway, I would have asked about the type of dementia education provided to the staff on a regular basis, and I would have asked for clear guidelines about when my mother would need to move (if she became incontinent, for example). At Greenway I would have followed my mother's care more closely, visited her more often, and insisted on being included in her care plan meetings on a regular basis. Again, with the help of a geriatric care manager, I would have recognized perhaps a year earlier than I did that Mom needed a higher level of assistance and stimulation than Greenway could provide, that she needed a dedicated "memory care" home such as Elm Haven. When Mom needed rehab, a geriatric care manager could have helped me navigate the rocky transitions from facility to facility.

In 2005, when my mother and I visited an elder care attorney to transfer the cottage to me and fill out her Health Care Proxy, Living Will, and Durable Power of Attorney, I would not have trusted the attorney to understand everything about planning for elder care. I would have met with a financial advisor. Even though I was not planning on selling the cottage at that point, I would have talked to an expert about what to do with the money if we did sell it (such as not depositing it into my mother's checking account). And then before—not after—I submitted Mom's voluminous Medicaid application to Social Services, I would have reviewed it with both the attorney and the financial advisor.

But this is the real world, not one inhabited by Super Daughters and Mega Caregivers, and I am left with my imperfect self and my very human regrets. By sharing my story I hope to make your journey a bit easier. Each of us brings our own personality, history, and values to caregiving, but common challenges remain. I'm hopeful that our new National Plan to Address Alzheimer's Disease (see Appendix J) will help by increasing public understanding of Alzheimer's and the need for specialized care, and that funding and answers will surface as more and more Americans fall prey to dementia.

In the summer of 2012, my mother continues to sit up in her wheelchair, smiling. Her health remains fairly stable and she eats well. Today though, as happens a few times per month, she suffers a seizure. I find her curled up in bed, staring into space, unresponsive. No one knows what causes them, though I'm told they're not unusual in people with advanced dementia. To me she seems so tiny and "gone," so much like the images I've seen of people in the last stage of Alzheimer's disease, that all I can do is stroke her hand and cry.

But by the end of our visit, Mom is sitting up, bright-eyed and smiling, drinking me in. She enjoys three pieces of chocolate, and smells the roses I brought. With the spell broken, we return to the present.

And so it goes. Each day brings loss; each day, recovery. A long journey, one day at a time.

Appendices

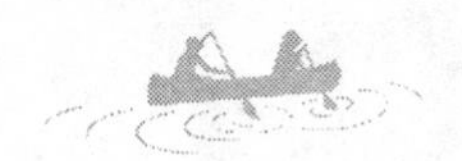

Appendix A: *Is There a Test to Diagnose Alzheimer's Disease?*

No test exists, as of this writing, that will confirm a diagnosis of Alzheimer's disease. Clinical trials looking at body fluids and imaging results show promise, but because they are still being evaluated and standardized, these tests are not yet available to primary care doctors.

However, doctors can diagnose "probable Alzheimer's disease" with 90% accuracy with neuropsychological testing and by ruling out other causes of memory problems and cognitive decline. A medical history can rule out depression; lab work can rule out urinary infection, thyroid dysfunction, and vitamin deficiencies; and a CT scan and MRI can rule out strokes, trauma and tumors.

PET Scans

According to Dr. Frank Longo, a Stanford University neuroscientist, two kinds of PET scans can be used to find evidence of probable Alzheimer's disease in the brain, although each is imperfect. The first can show decreased levels of metabolic activity, but it's not accurate enough to use for diagnosis. The second is an amyloid PET scan, in which an intravenous injection of florbetapir, a radioactive drug approved by the Food and Drug Administration in April 2012, binds to amyloid plaques. Amyloid PET scans show plaques on 96% of people with severe Alzheimer's disease and two-thirds of those with mild cognitive impairment. Longo says this tool may be available to primary care doctors by the summer of 2012, but it's unlikely to be covered by Medicare at first. And he cautions that one-third of people aged 65 and over exhibiting normal cognition also show amyloid plaques on these PET scans—and they may never develop Alzheimer's disease. The Alzheimer's Association reserves judgment on this new tool, since "a positive scan...has limited utility at this point. Having amyloid buildup in your brain does not mean for certain that you have Alzheimer's disease." They recommend further research into the use of such PET imaging.

Spinal Fluid Tests

A spinal fluid test has been approved for use that identifies the presence of certain markers of Alzheimer's disease—the proteins beta amyloid and tau—but it cannot accurately predict who will develop Alzheimer's disease. Research on this spinal test showed that among the test subjects with Alzheimer's disease, a huge percentage—ninety percent—had high levels of these proteins in their spinal fluid, but among those with mild cognitive impairment, only seventy-two percent had the markers. However, thirty-six percent of those with no symptoms of dementia still had the markers. If we want to test people before they develop symptoms of the disease, or to catch the disease early, the spinal fluid test is not accurate enough to be definitive. Many doctors and researchers are reluctant to recommend this test as it cannot confirm a diagnosis, and no treatments exist.

Biomarkers

In May of 2011, an international workgroup of more than forty top Alzheimer's researchers, organized by the Alzheimer's Association and the National Institute on Aging (NIA) of the National Institutes of Health, published new criteria and guidelines for the diagnosis of Alzheimer's disease—the first time the criteria and guidelines had been updated in 27 years. To make such a diagnosis, they argue, it's not enough to rely simply on observing a person's behavior or to conduct a neuropsychological exam. Alzheimer's research must find specific biochemical substances in the body that mark the presence or absence of the disease or that reveal the risk of developing the disease ("biomarkers"). Research must prove the value of those biomarkers, and it must assure the medical community that all diagnostic tests using those biomarkers will offer reliable results and remain consistent from one laboratory to another. That's a tall order, and the committee acknowledges that it may take ten years or more for scientists to identify the correct biomarkers.

For now, the workgroup calls for intensive research on two types of biomarkers: the level of beta-amyloid in the brain, and damage or degeneration of nerve cells. Beta amyloid blocks the transmission of nerve impulses, and many researchers now agree that smaller beta amyloid particles, if not the larger plaques themselves, play a major role in the development of Alzheimer's disease.

These smaller bits of amyloid beta build up in the brain years before plaques are formed or a patient receives a diagnosis of Alzheimer's disease, and slowly kill the brain. Tests on mice show that the substance that eventually turns into amyloid plaques—amyloid precursor protein, or APP—causes the death of olfactory nerve cells, which are closely related to brain cells. (Loss of the sense of smell is one symptom of Alzheimer's disease.) This degeneration starts not on the outside of the cells with larger plaques, as previously assumed, but inside the cells with this smaller amyloid substance. Dr. Jack Diamond, the scientific director at the Alzheimer Society of Canada, says that "by the time the plaques are formed, all the damage to the nerve cells has been done. A successful treatment would have to affect the amyloid molecules, not the plaques themselves."

• • •

Re-defining the Stages of Alzheimer's Disease

The international workgroup mentioned above also recommends that the stages of Alzheimer's be revised to include the many years—perhaps decades—before any symptoms occur. They call this lengthy stage "preclinical Alzheimer's disease." When I read this, I find it frightening to think that Alzheimer's could be stalking my own brain right this moment, while I am in my forties. Researchers and doctors cannot say for sure what is normal aging and what is preclinical Alzheimer's disease. I already know that I am high-risk, with a mother who has dementia and shows so many symptoms of Alzheimer's. The international workgroup calls for more research into the biomarkers of this first stage, to help us recognize, diagnose, and treat it before any decline occurs.

I hope that in ten years the pages I'm writing here on Alzheimer's research will be obsolete, that we will know how to prevent, treat, and cure Alzheimer's disease and other dementias. For the moment, though, I continue to discover in my reading more promising—if sometimes conflicting—trends in Alzheimer's research. As Diamond points out, "We're now at a crossroads....Some of the things that we always assumed are now no longer acceptable as fully explaining the disease."

Appendix B
Medications Approved to Relieve Symptoms of Alzheimer's Disease

Two types of prescription medications have been approved by the FDA to treat the symptoms of Alzheimer's disease. They are not a cure, and while they may lessen the symptoms of the disease, they will not slow its progression.

As enzyme blockers, the first group—the cholinesterase inhibitors—work by restoring the balance of neurotransmitters in the brain. They include Aricept (donepezil HCl), approved by the FDA in 1993; Exelon (rivastigmine), approved in 1997; and Razadyne (galantamine), approved in 2001. Exelon and Razadyne are approved for mild to moderate dementia, and Aricept is approved for mild to severe dementia.

The second type of medication is an N-methyl D-aspartate (NMDA) antagonist. Namenda (memantine), approved in 2003, can delay progression of some symptoms in moderate to severe cases of Alzheimer's disease. It regulates glutamate, an important brain chemical.

There is evidence that a combination of these two types of medications—Namenda plus a cholinesterase inhibitor—is more effective at relieving the symptoms of Alzheimer's disease than treatment with only one type. A two-and-a-half-year study by the Memory Disorder Unit at Massachusetts General Hospital, published in 2008, showed that test subjects with mild dementia who took a combination of these drugs experienced a slower decline in memory and function than test subjects who took one type of medication or a placebo. A study published in the *Journal of the American Medical Association* in 2004 showed similar results with patients with moderate to severe dementia; when those already taking a cholinesterase inhibitor added Namenda, they experienced more of an increase in cognitive function and ability to perform activities of daily living than those solely on a cholinesterase inhibitor. Those on combination therapy also experienced a lower rate of side effects, especially gastrointestinal issues.

Appendix C: Risk Factors and Antidotes for Dementia

As a large French multi-center task force states in their report, *Prevention of Progression to Dementia in the Elderly*, "our present state of knowledge is inadequate."

None of us know if the health dictates we follow to avoid dementia will turn out in thirty years to have been bad advice. Mom taught me, for example, to avoid butter, to buy margarine because it didn't have cholesterol (and because it was cheaper), but now the public knows about trans fat, and I wonder if that margarine and all the store-bought cookies she ate loaded her arteries with trans fat and contributed to her small strokes and dementia. (A 2011 study published by the journal *Neurology* shows a strong correlation between trans fat in the bloodstream and decreased brain function.)

Most scientists agree, however, that there are certain risk factors for Alzheimer's disease. They include old age; a family history; serious head trauma; poor cardiovascular health; high blood pressure; stroke; diabetes; high cholesterol; obesity in middle age; a low education level (which predisposes someone to less learning and brain development over their lifetime); and smoking.

Exercise

Some researchers say that exercise may be our most powerful antidote for Alzheimer's disease. Because aerobic exercise increases blood flow to the brain, stimulates the growth of new brain cells, and decreases the risk of heart attack, stroke, and diabetes, the Alzheimer's Association recommends thirty minutes of daily exercise.

A recent study by neurologists at Rush University Medical Center shows that daily activity of all kinds—from formal exercise to activities such as washing dishes, cleaning, and cooking—may reduce the risk of developing Alzheimer's disease, even in people over age 80. In another study, subjects who walked forty minutes a day for a year regained volume in their hippocampus, reversing brain shrinkage. In a third study, people with mild cognitive impairment who did resistance weight training two times a week over six months showed an increase in their memory and executive function (the ability to multi-task).

Mental Stimulation

Social activity and mental stimulation are also crucial. Combining social activity and mental stimulation with regular exercise is more effective than doing only one or the other. Sports, cultural activities, emotional support, and close personal relationships are all key. We should work as long as we can, volunteer, join social clubs, and travel. We should turn off the television, read, write, do crosswords and puzzles. Play games, do memory exercises, learn a new language, or learn to play an instrument. In fact, if we challenge ourselves regularly, our brains will continue to create new cells and connections.

In the last ten years Mom lived at the cottage, she had little social interaction, scant mental stimulation beyond reading, and no exercise beyond climbing the hill to her car once or twice a week in winter.

My life in an intentional community is quite different. I can hike with a friend through our fields, work with a team to cook a village meal, or play an instrument and perform skits in our village talent shows. There's always something to do, and someone to do it with.

The Role of Diet

The Alzheimer's Association recommends a low-fat, low-cholesterol diet, but acknowledges that all cholesterol is not the same: research suggests that HDL, or "good" cholesterol, may help protect brain cells. They recommend lots of dark vegetables and fruits that are high in antioxidants; mono- or polyunsaturated fats such as olive oil, cold water fish high in Omega 3's (salmon, tuna, mackerel); and nuts such as almonds, pecans, and walnuts. Vitamin E, or vitamin E and C together, vitamin B12, and folate may also decrease the risk of Alzheimer's.

In 2005, when Mom lived with us, I barely had time to think of my own health. Not only was I seriously overweight, but I was insulin resistant and pre-diabetic and didn't know it yet. (Insulin in the blood delivers glucose—blood sugar—to the body's cells. With insulin resistance and pre-diabetes, cells grow resistant to the insulin, too much glucose remains in the blood and damages organs, and then the pancreas pumps out even more insulin to force the cells to absorb the glucose. If the pancreas grows exhausted and stops producing enough insulin, you get Type II diabetes.) I had also become quite allergic for the first time in my life to pollen, dust, and wheat, and was prone to frequent attacks of bronchitis.

Gradually, over the past few years, while a variety of facilities have taken on the care of Mom's daily physical needs, I have paid more attention to my own. I've lost weight and lowered my blood sugar level on a low-carbohydrate, wheat-free, sugar-free diet under the supervision of a nutritionist. I get shots every two weeks for my allergies, and garden, walk, and swim for exercise. I'm no longer felled by bronchitis, and rarely get sick.

• • •

The Importance of Vision Screening

Research has found a connection between vision and Alzheimer's disease. In a study of elderly people over the age of 71, all of whom had normal cognitive functioning at the beginning of the study, those who had undiagnosed or untreated vision problems showed a 9.5-fold increase in the risk of developing Alzheimer's disease.

Unfortunately, Medicare Parts A and B do not cover routine vision screenings, only a yearly exam for those at high risk for glaucoma. In France, a dementia task force recommends that vision screening be included in all evaluations to prevent Alzheimer's.

Sleep Apnea and Dementia

I'm also getting treatment for sleep apnea, which I never knew I had. One day a few months ago, I was doing a relaxation meditation lying down, near the edge of sleep, and I felt the tissues of my throat close up and my breathing cut off. For several years, I've been exhausted all day despite nine or ten hours of sleep, but if it weren't for my meditation practice I might never have discovered the sleep apnea. My husband is such a sound sleeper he never noticed if I snored a lot, or if I stopped breathing and startled awake. My only symptoms, aside from extreme fatigue, were frequent headaches first thing in the morning.

The hospital's sleep clinic discovered that I stop breathing up to twenty times an hour. With sleep apnea, you wake up partially over and over, but you don't remember waking up. Now I use a Continuous Positive Airway Pressure (CPAP) machine each night, a mask over my nose and mouth that pumps a stream of air into my throat to keep the tissues from collapsing. I wake refreshed, and throughout the day my energy stays constant.

I suspect that my mother also has sleep apnea. Years ago, before I married, I'd visit her and sleep in the extra twin bed in her bedroom. She sounded like a chainsaw revved and turned off, revved and turned off. Every few minutes her loud, rumbling snores would stop, and after a moment she would snort, as if catching her breath, and continue snoring. She snored at our house, too. She had never been tested for sleep apnea, and at this point she wouldn't be able to wear a CPAP mask without tugging it off.

After a few months of feeling better on the CPAP, I researched the condition online. A study led by the University of California, San Francisco, shows that elderly women who have sleep apnea are about twice as likely to develop dementia as those without the condition. Other researchers find that people whose nightly sleep is short or disturbed have higher levels of beta amyloid, the protein that causes plaques between brain cells. According to a study at the Washington University School of Medicine in St. Louis, in younger people, or older people who sleep well, excess beta amyloid drains out of their brains during sleep into their spinal fluid. Dr. Stephen Duntley, professor of neurology and director of Washington University's Sleep Medicine Center, says, "It's still speculation, but there are tantalizing hints that better sleep may be helpful in reducing Alzheimer's disease risk."

Is Damage Reversible?

In 2010, researchers in Milan, Italy, found that CPAP therapy can restore brain tissue in people with sleep apnea. Before treatment, the subjects had less gray matter volume than normal, but after three months on a CPAP machine their gray matter had increased significantly. Restored gray matter in specific hippocampal and frontal brain regions can improve executive functioning (cognitive abilities such as planning, verbal reasoning, problem-solving, and multi-tasking) and short-term memory. The lead researcher, Vincenza Castronovo, Ph.D., a clinical psychologist and psychotherapist, states in an article in Science Daily that not only does gray matter increase with CPAP treatment, but "neuropsychological deficits are reversed."

My mother's neuropsychological exam in 1997 showed mildly slowed executive functioning, diminished sustained attention, and mild word finding difficulties. I wish that the doctors had asked her about her snoring and her day-time fatigue. There's no mention in their report of her odd sleeping patterns—the difficulty sleeping at night, the napping half the day. Not only could sleep apnea have explained these patterns, and killed off some of her gray matter, it would have exacerbated all of the other health problems that put her at risk for Alzheimer's—her high blood pressure, depression, and small strokes.

We know that the obese have a higher rate of sleep apnea than people of normal weight, but research shows that slim people who sit for many hours a day—office workers and truck drivers, for example—are also at risk. My mother carried extra weight in her fifties and sixties, and sat for many hours a day at her desk the last ten years she lived at the cottage. (As a writer, I also sit a lot, of course, but I try to take a break every hour to move around.) The Sleep Research Laboratory of the Toronto Rehabilitation Institute has found that, in men of normal weight who sit for hours, fluid builds up in their legs during the day, and then, at night in bed, shifts to their necks. The fluid reduces the size of their airways and increases the likelihood of tissue collapse.

The National Sleep Foundation estimates that more than 18 million American adults have sleep apnea. According to the American Sleep Apnea Association, sleep apnea is as common as Type II diabetes, but "because of the lack of awareness by the public and health care professionals, the vast majority of sleep apnea patients remain undiagnosed and therefore untreated."

CPAP machines have been widely available since the late 1980s. Perhaps if doctors had suggested to my mother years ago that she be evaluated at a sleep clinic, perhaps if she had started to wear a CPAP machine in the early stages of her dementia, its progression could have been slowed.

Hope in Vaccines?

Vaccines to reduce the build-up of these amyloid molecules are now being tested in more than 40 clinical trials with approximately 20,000 people. Similar trials in 2000 resulted in the death of two people from inflammation of the brain, and even though autopsies showed that the plaques had been reduced, their dementia had continued unabated. Diamond says, "if we stop the amyloid from accumulating, it doesn't mean we've found the cure we need."

Other studies are being conducted to create a vaccine for the tau protein tangles that form inside nerve cells. Some say that cognitive decline really starts when tau protein, not amyloid, builds up, damaging nerve cells.

Startling new research in February, 2012, shows that tau plays a major role in the spread of Alzheimer's disease in the brain, proving in studies with genetically-engineered mice that Alzheimer's disease originates in one particular area behind the ears, the entorhinal cortex (where memories are created and stored), and that it spreads like an infection to neighboring parts of the brain. This research, conducted separately in independent studies at Columbia and Harvard Universities, shows that broken, tangled tau protein in one neuron somehow causes tau in adjacent neurons to break down and develop tangles. The mice were genetically engineered to make human tau protein only in their entorhinal cortex, and in no other areas of their brain. When that human tau protein began to break and tangle, and then appeared in adjacent areas of their brain, it was clear for the first time that broken tau does not develop sporadically in more susceptible parts of the brain (what has been called the "bad neighborhood" hypothesis), but is passed from neuron to neuron.

These findings offer the tantalizing possibility that there may be a way to stop Alzheimer's disease by preventing broken tau protein from "infecting" its neighbors. However, it remains unclear how tau and amyloid beta work together, and scientists warn that any treatment or antibody based on this tau research would require many more years of study, and significant funding.

Appendix D:
Is It "All in the Family"?

In Familial (early-onset) Alzheimer's, gene mutations cause a cascade of effects in the brain leading to increased amyloid. If one parent carries the mutated gene, the child has a fifty percent chance of developing the disease; if both parents carry the gene, the risk increases to seventy-five percent.

In Alzheimer's disease over age sixty, there is something called a "risk factor" gene—APOE ε4 allele. This gene increases your risk somewhat if you inherit it from your parents. According to the National Institute on Aging, "Some people with one or two APOEε4 alleles never get the disease, and others who develop Alzheimer's do not have any APOEε4 alleles." For that reason a blood test for the allele is not recommended for people at risk for Alzheimer's disease.

Because of my mother's breast cancer in her forties, I did have the blood test done for the gene that would place me at higher risk for breast cancer (I don't have it), but for this Alzheimer's risk factor gene I'm unlikely, for the reasons above, to get a blood test. I consider myself fortunate that I've learned as much as I have in my forties about Alzheimer's disease, and that through prevention and self-education, I may be able to avoid many of the risk factors.

Appendix E: The Role of Infection

New and on-going Alzheimer's research ranges widely over many branches of inquiry: stem cell treatments, "growth factors" to repair damage to nerve cells, the damage caused by free radicals, the role of stress in cell damage (glucocorticoids such as cortisol may cause insulin resistance), and infection.

To look at just one of these subjects—infection—researchers know that parasites, bacteria, and viruses in the central nervous system can excrete toxins and cause inflammation, which in turn damage neurons. People with cold sores, from the herpes virus HSVI, are more likely to develop Alzheimer's. (Mom and I both get cold sores.) Other viruses connected with Alzheimer's risk are the herpes virus that produces the roseola rash, HIV, hepatitis C, and cytomegalovirus. Research into bacteria shows that people with Alzheimer's have more spirochetes in their brains, which infect neurons. When Chlamydia pneumoniae, a common cause of pneumonia, is injected into mouse brains, they develop amyloid plaques.

Appendix F:
Sweet Poison: The Toxic Tide of Sugar

As I watch my mother's deterioration I have become more determined to prevent my own.

After I discovered that I have sleep apnea—a risk factor for dementia—I found more evidence in my research that sleep apnea may be tied to insulin resistance and pre-diabetes, and to Alzheimer's disease. During sleep, insulin levels in the body normally decline, but if the sleep is disrupted, insulin levels remain high. High insulin has been connected to inflammation in many parts of the body, including the brain, and inflammation puts a person at risk for stroke and heart disease, among other things. Our brains produce insulin independent of that produced in the pancreas, but if there is too much insulin it seems to increase the amount of amyloid beta. Also, a study at the University of Pittsburgh Medical Center determined that the brains of mice subjected to intermittent periods of low oxygen, as with sleep apnea, showed less sensitivity to insulin. (However, if the mice were consistently subject to a low oxygen level, as when people hike at high elevations, there was no change in their insulin sensitivity.) We need more research on the relationship of sleep apnea to metabolic disorders such as insulin resistance, pre-diabetes, and diabetes.

Many researchers now describe Alzheimer's disease as "Type III diabetes," diabetes of the brain. Researchers have known for some time that people with Type II diabetes are twice as likely as those without diabetes to develop Alzheimer's. Diabetics on insulin therapy are four times as likely as non-diabetics to develop Alzheimer's. The worldwide epidemic of Alzheimer's disease has grown alongside the worldwide epidemic of Type II diabetes. Someone like me who is insulin resistant and pre-diabetic is 70% more likely than someone with normal blood sugar and insulin levels to develop Alzheimer's disease. We do not need to be fully diabetic to raise our risk considerably. Being overweight or obese, or having a lot of belly fat in middle age (as I do, and my mother did), are often related to insulin resistance and increase the risk of dementia.

I think of all the years my mother ate large amounts of sugar—when she stopped drinking, the pound bags of M&M's; over the last years at the cottage, tons of cookies and ice cream. Although she was never diagnosed with diabetes, it's likely that, like me, Mom has been pre-diabetic and insulin-resistant for years.

While twenty million people in the United States have Type II diabetes, twice that number are insulin resistant and pre-diabetic. Unfortunately, this condition often goes undiagnosed until it progresses into full-blown diabetes. With so many of us pre-diabetic, we need more awareness of this condition, and more research into its connection to Alzheimer's.

In 2010, researchers at Kyushu University in Japan reported that people with diabetes or pre-diabetes are more likely to develop beta amyloid brain plaques. Another study has determined that a nasal spray of insulin improves the brain's use of glucose, as well as memory and cognitive functioning. Some anti-diabetic drugs, such as rosiglitazone, seem to help brain functioning in people with Alzheimer's.

A team at Northwestern University has determined that a toxic protein, called an ADDL (amyloid beta-derived diffusible ligand), strips brain nerve cells of insulin receptors, leaving them insulin resistant. Both brain insulin and its receptors are lower in people with Alzheimer's disease. ADDL's start to build up at the beginning of Alzheimer's disease, but may prove to be reversible.

Low-Carb Diets for the Brain

For the past year I've slowly eaten less and less sugar and starch—down, now, to less than 30 mg a day, mostly from vegetables; I eat primarily animal fat and protein (organic whenever I can), raw cheese, eggs, olive oil, and low-carb vegetables. When I started this diet I didn't know about the connection between insulin sensitivity and neuron damage. I wanted simply to lose weight and to lower my high blood sugar level so I wouldn't develop diabetes; in the past, a less drastic reduction in carbohydrates had not worked for me. For my whole adult life I'd followed the general medical advice since the 1980s to eat low fat—which essentially means high-carbohydrate—and by my mid-thirties I carried the extra eighty pounds I mentioned earlier.

With this low-carb diet I hope to move my metabolism from glucose-based and insulin resistant to something called "ketonic" or "ketogenic." When our bodies, including our brains, run on fat, not glucose, we're using ketones for energy, which is perfectly healthy and efficient. In fact, a product called Axona® has been shown in a recent study to improve the cognitive functioning of some people with Alzheimer's disease by overcoming their brains' resistance to glucose by fueling them with ketones. A prescription, FDA-designated "medical food," Axona is a powder mixed with water or food and consumed once a day. According to Accera, the maker of Axona, "Ketone bodies are naturally occurring compounds that are produced mainly by the liver from fatty acids during periods of extended fasting. Ketone bodies have been demonstrated to protect neurons."

Several families in my heavily-vegetarian community have also switched in recent years, for different reasons, to low-carb or high-fat ketogenic diets: "paleo" diets based on a hunter-gatherer diet, before agriculture, with organic meat, fish, vegetables, small amounts of fruit, roots, and nuts; "Gut and Psychology Syndrome ("GAPS") diets heavy on organic fatty meat, soups made from bones, fish, eggs, butter, fermented vegetables, nuts, seeds, coconut, and olive oil; and low-carb diets based on the recommendations of the Weston A. Price Foundation that studies the food and health of "traditional" societies around the world. Several of us buy whole, raw milk from a neighbor's cow, delivered weekly; we enjoy organic, free-range eggs, with their rich, orange yolks, from a local farmer and from coops in our own backyards; and this fall we expect another delivery of organic, grass-fed beef—affordable purchased in bulk—from another neighbor with a large herd of pastured dairy cattle.

I follow the advice of Gary Taubes in his book *Good Calories, Bad Calories: Challenging the Conventional Wisdom on Diet, Weight Control, and Disease* (and his shorter version of the book, *Why We Get Fat, and What to Do About It*). I eat very little grain, legumes or fruit, and supplement our family's meat-based diet with my large vegetable garden. My diet is low in the inflammatory Omega 6's so prevalent in grain, processed foods, and vegetable oils, and rich in anti-inflammatory Omega 3's. Though my total cholesterol level is higher than most doctors consider optimal, it is not primarily LDL, the "bad," low-density kind that forms plaque on arterial walls, but mostly HDL, the high-density, fluffy kind that is less likely to clump and cause stroke and heart disease. Even on a diet high in animal fat, my triglycerides—a risk factor for stroke and heart attack—continue to go down.

Although I don't pay attention to most bloggers on medical issues (and refer in this book only to research published by established medical associations), I do follow the blog of Dr. Emily Deans, a psychiatrist who believes in "evolutionary medicine"—how "diseases of civilization...are caused by differences between our current lives and our evolutionary suitability, and that replicating a hunter-gatherer life in many ways (as makes scientific and practical sense) can lead to better health, both physical and mental." Referring to the connection between glucose, insulin, amyloid build-up, and Alzheimer's, she says, "if you wanted to stop Alzheimer's by targeting amyloid, you would have to start decades earlier [before plaques form]...Low-carbers, paleo diet enthusiasts...or anyone else who avoids hyperglycemia could be preventing amyloid build-up at this long prodromal stage, thus possibly reducing risk of later Alzheimer's."

It's all supposition at this point, but for someone like me who has insulin resistance, a ketogenic diet may be a good idea. Starting now, I may be able to prevent insulin resistance in my brain, and a concomitant build-up of amyloid beta.

Appendix G: The Benefits of "Memory Consultations" and Early Diagnosis

Memory Consultations

Countries such as France are ahead of us in providing "memory consultations." A French multi-center task force recommends a comprehensive memory consultation for every elder on a regular basis—with an initial consultation before they experience memory or cognitive decline.

The consultation would evaluate areas such as nutrition, metabolic functioning (diabetes, insulin resistance, etc.), depression, activities of daily living, gait and balance, frailty, age, sex, education, living arrangements, medical history, a clinical examination, and cognitive functioning. These evaluations would involve a general practitioner, geriatrician, and a neurologist—not one or two, but all three.

Memory care programs in the United States offer similar consultations with multi-disciplinary teams, but as the website of the Memory Care Program at the University of Rochester Medical Center points out, "One of the barriers to creating a comprehensive memory care program is that...while health insurance covers some aspects of dementia care, many of the important time-intensive evaluations and follow-up care services are not reimbursed." We have excellent memory care programs, but access may be limited.

• • •

Wellness Visits

As of January 2011, under the Affordable Care Act, anyone with Medicare Part B is eligible for an annual wellness visit that includes a cognitive assessment, an evaluation of risk factors for diseases such as Alzheimer's, and recommendations for referrals to programs to help reduce those risk factors (such as seeing a nutritionist or joining a smoking cessation program). This annual visit, which is fully covered with no deductible, co-insurance, or co-payment, and thus helps seniors who cannot afford to go to the doctor until they're ill, is a step in the right direction.

According to the Centers for Medicare & Medicaid Services, however, by the end of 2011 only an estimated 1.3 million people will have received a wellness exam, out of the 46 million who are eligible. Whatever the reasons for the program's under-utilization, I can't help but think that if my mother had had access to annual wellness visits under Medicare from the age of 65, with its cognitive assessment and discussion of her risk factors, she might have changed some habits and been in better health over the following ten years.

Benefits of Early Diagnosis

Many doctors—including my mother's small-town family doctor and Dr. Claiborne—shy away from a diagnosis of Alzheimer's, but a recent survey by the Harvard School of Public Health, of adults in France, Germany, Poland, Spain, and the United States, indicates that most people want to know as soon as possible if they're showing signs of Alzheimer's. Contrary to what one might expect, they don't want to hide from the possibility; they want early diagnosis so they have a shot, however minor, at prevention and delay.

In their 2011 report *Alzheimer's Disease Facts and Figures*, the Alzheimer's Association explains why early detection and diagnosis is so crucial. The list is long, but worth sharing:

a) The cognitive decline may be caused by something treatable, such as depression or a vitamin B12 deficiency, and early diagnosis prevents further decline;
b) It's important to discuss the diagnosis with family members and begin the search for appropriate support services;
c) Such a discussion reduces anxiety by naming the problem;
d) Medication and other approaches may be used to manage symptoms;
e) Early diagnosis gives people the option of joining clinical trials;
f) It allows more awareness of how some combinations of medications make symptoms worse;
g) It alerts doctors and family members to the possibility that the person may need assistance with daily tasks such as cooking and managing medications;
h) It may reduce falls and other accidents because caregivers are more aware of the dangers;
i) It allows an awareness of financial problems such as the person giving money to scams; and
j) It allows the person with dementia and their family members to plan for the future.

I can't help but wonder how the last years of my mother's life at the cottage—and the seven years since then—might have been different if she'd received a diagnosis of mixed dementia years ago. If she'd been given a comprehensive, written evaluation, she would have studied it thoroughly. Most likely, the weight of its authority would have prompted her to share it with me.

Appendix H: Planning for Long-Term Care

When I think of my own financial future with Ben, and the astronomical cost of long-term care, my gut reaction, like that of many Americans, is to say, "Why bother saving every penny for our old age? Why bother saving anything?" The only thing that will convince me to plan ahead for long-term care is if we can invest in affordable, guaranteed long-term care insurance.

In March of 2010, President Obama signed a bill passed by Congress called the Community Living Assistance Services and Supports (CLASS) Act, to provide the first national long-term care insurance program in the United States—the kind of program most developed nations already have. CLASS was designed to help people with disabilities or cognitive impairment who need help with activities of daily living (ADLs) such as bathing, dressing, and eating, and who want to remain at home and stay out of a nursing home, and also to relieve the burden on family caregivers. Benefits could be applied not only to in-home care but to adult day care in the community, assisted living, and nursing homes.

By the fall of 2011, though, CLASS was revoked. Not enough young, healthy people were expected to enroll and keep the program afloat. An amendment also required that the program be proven to be financially self-sustaining for 75 years, and that could not be assured. Robert Yee, the program's chief actuary, said that the program might have worked if the waiting period before receiving benefits were expanded from five to fifteen years, and if the program had started only with large employers.

If CLASS had existed successfully years ago as it's written now, my mother would have been required to pay the premiums for at least five years before receiving benefits. She would have been required to enroll while she was still working at least part-time, and to work for at least three years of the five before she could receive benefits. (If your employer participates, you can opt out of the automatic deduction, thus making it voluntary.) In my mother's case she would have had to enroll by her mid-50s.

Premiums for CLASS average $123 a month, which is $1476 a year—less for younger people, and more for older people. This amount would have been a prudent investment for most people, if the Act had survived, as at least seventy percent of people over age 65 need chronic long-term care services that are not covered by Medicare (or by Medicaid until after they've spent their savings and become impoverished). Forty percent of people receiving chronic long-term care are between the ages of 18 and 64, often because of sudden injury or illness such as a head injury or stroke.

We are all likely to need long-term care at some point. According to the Family Caregiver Alliance, "the lifetime probability of becoming disabled in at least two different activities of daily living or of becoming cognitively impaired is 68% for people age 65 and older." While three out of ten elders will die quickly and never need long-term care, and seventeen percent of elders will need assistance for only a year or less, more than fifty percent will need help for at least a year. One out of five elders will need assistance for five years or more. Women are twice as likely as men to need care for more than five years.

Long-term care at home lasts an average of three to five years, assisted living care 2.5 to 3 years, and nursing home care 2.3 years. Twenty percent of people age sixty-five will end up spending over

$100,000 in long-term care costs, and one in twenty will spend more than $250,000. Despite these statistics (odds much less in our favor than, say, the odds that we'll burn down our house and need homeowners insurance), few of us buy private long-term care insurance—less than 3 percent.

One benefit of CLASS, compared to private long-term care insurance companies, was that no one could be excluded from enrollment because of a pre-existing condition—even a diagnosis of Alzheimer's disease. That's not to be underestimated.

If CLASS had existed years ago and my mother had paid the premiums, she would have been able to receive benefits—mandated to be at least $50 a day, and estimated to be an average of $75 a day—when she first needed assistance or supervision with activities of daily living after she was injured in assisted living. In fact, triggers for benefits in CLASS included any cognitive impairment that lasts for at least 90 days and requires assistance or supervision for health and safety, so Mom might have qualified for aides at the cottage or in my home, as she needed help to cook and clean.

My mother's savings ran out two years into her stay at Elm Haven, so if CLASS had paid for half of her care for those two years, and part of the cost of private aides and assisted living before that, she could have lived at Elm Haven for at least four years instead of two (if her health allowed). Ben and I might not have had to sell the cottage.

If the CLASS Act had continued, Ben and I would have participated in it. In the absence of such a public program, I know we should buy private long-term care insurance, but the cost will be a stretch, and we will put it off.

According to Howard Gleckman, author of the book *Caring for Our Parents*, the best time to purchase private long-term care insurance in the United States is in your fifties, when the premiums are more affordable. Since Ben and I can't afford premiums now, we will hedge our bets that we will make it to our mid-fifties without a serious pre-existing condition that would disqualify us for acceptance. (If we are unlucky, and suspect that one of us has early dementia, we will try to make sure that we secure long-term care insurance *before* we ask a doctor for a diagnosis and it's recorded in our medical files.)

The average annual premium for private long-term care insurance for a fifty-year-old is about $850. For that you get a higher average daily benefit rate than with CLASS—$100 instead of $75; four years of coverage; and 5% compounded inflation protection, which is very important, because without inflation protection a policy is worthless. The average annual premium rises at age 65 to $1,800, at 79 to $5,500.

Private long-term care insurance needs more government regulation to be viable and affordable. Other countries have public long-term care insurance programs that work. Germany, for example, collects premiums for long-term care as a payroll deduction, much like our Medicare and Social Security, through a person's entire life, making the premiums affordable for everyone. The deductions, 1.95 percent of wages in 2008, are mandatory, not optional as in our CLASS Act, but Germans consider them to be not a tax, as Americans would, but as insurance, much as we all insure our homes and our cars. The funds from these premiums are held and invested not by the German government, which might be tempted to spend them, as our government would, but by a quasi-private company. German long-term care insurance covers both home and institutional care and benefits can be received in cash. Their premium deductions may need to double by 2040 to cover costs, but overall the system works well, and ninety percent of Germans receiving benefits report that they are satisfied.

Britain, on the other hand, has a system much like ours, with

Medicaid-like government funds supporting those who do not have private long-term care insurance and who run out of savings. Neither the British system nor ours will survive the "silver tsunami" without significant change. Gleckman writes that "the United States is quietly heading for a financial, medical, and social meltdown…It is hard to imagine what is about to happen, not just to millions of individual families, but to our nation. It will profoundly change tens of millions of lives, ruin carefully planned retirements, and profoundly alter the way we think of our government."

In the United States, a small but mandatory payroll deduction for a public long-term care insurance program would go a long way toward preventing that meltdown. If everyone had long-term care insurance, Medicaid would cease to be the fallback long-term care insurance program for millions of older Americans. The federal government and the states would be released from the catastrophic burden of Medicaid spending for elder care; the system could focus again on its original, and much less costly, intention from the 1960s—to aid poor women and children.

As the boomers enter late old age—when, again, fifty percent of those over age 85 have Alzheimer's disease—public long-term care insurance could mean the difference between government solvency and implosion.

Appendix I:
Long-Term Care in an Intentional Community

With long-term care insurance, Ben and I would be more likely to be able to continue to live at home in our intentional community if one or both of us became disabled. If one of us becomes the primary caregiver for the other, we will be able to afford some home care assistance to give the caregiver much needed respite. We know that, even though we live in community, our neighbors are too busy with their work and children to volunteer many hours of companionship, let alone offer hands-on care.

Even in elder cohousing, a relatively new kind of intentional community where residents are all 50 or older, few people are willing to offer daily hands-on assistance with activities of daily living (ADLs) such as bathing, dressing and toileting. In his book *Senior Cohousing: A Community Approach to Independent Living*, Charles Durrett writes about elder cohousing in Denmark, where it is well established, and in the United States, where it is growing in popularity. He says that "people will only give the type and amount of care that they feel like giving...Most residents just want to be neighbors, after all, not health aides." Usually the help they are willing to give will fill the gap before family members can arrange additional help, and allow the person who needs assistance to live in their home longer than they could if they didn't live in cohousing.

Ben and I expect that, like our neighbor Rita, if we need regular hands-on assistance, we will need to hire private aides. We hope that if others in our community need help with ADLs that we could share the cost. Durrett describes how some cohousing communities in Europe hire a resident nurse or nursing student to live in a studio apartment in their Common House. The nurse becomes a true member of the community, eating with the residents, sharing their celebrations and sorrows. When it comes time for a resident to need help, the hope would be that the nurse would treat them with true affection and respect. As long as we need help with at least two ADLs, or we need assistance or supervision because of a cognitive impairment, long-term care insurance might cover some of the cost of a shared nurse.

If either Ben or I—or both of us—must move to a facility offsite to get the care we need, good long-term care insurance coverage would protect us from impoverishment. We hope. Private long-term care insurance in the United States is a considerable gamble.

Appendix J: Confronting the Epidemic at the National Level and Beyond

Research Funding

Along with early diagnosis, affordable care for those who have dementia, and more assistance for family caregivers, we need an immediate increase in research funding. According to the Alzheimer's Association, "For every dollar the government spends on the costs of Alzheimer care, it invests less than a penny in research to find a cure." In their May 2011 report *Penny Wise, Pound Foolish: Fairness and Funding at the National Institute on Aging*, the Alzheimer's Foundation of America, a coalition of over 1,600 organizations, warns of a "substantial risk that geriatric researchers will move on to other areas of science with greater prospects of funding...If the NIA [the National Institute on Aging, part of NIH] funding is not significantly increased, we stand to lose a generation or more of young and emerging investigators in aging and Alzheimer's disease." The AFA quotes Sam Gandy, M.D., Ph.D., Professor of Neurology and Psychiatry, Mount Sinai Chair in Alzheimer's Disease Research, and Associate Director, Mount Sinai Alzheimer's Disease Research Center:

> "We can no longer, in good conscience, recommend that our trainees plan for a career in Alzheimer's research unless they can establish their first labs in China, Korea, Europe, Australia, or South America."

In February 2012, the Obama administration announced an immediate increase in the federal budget of $50 million for Alzheimer's research, with $80 million added for the fiscal year 2013 budget. An additional $26 million will help provide community support for family caregivers, improve the training of health care providers, and raise public awareness.

I'm excited by the funding for family caregivers and public awareness of the disease, but I doubt that this increase in research funding will make a difference. Many experts agree. Consider the fact that, in 2011, the federal government allotted only $450 million for Alzheimer's research through the National Institutes of Health, compared to over $3 billion for HIV/AIDs, over $4 billion for heart and cardiovascular disease, and nearly $6 billion for cancer. An addition of $130 million over two years would bring the total for Alzheimer's research to only $580 million—a paltry sum. Unless this imbalance is corrected—unless we agree as a nation to fund a wide spectrum of research, over many years, in hundreds of laboratories—we are unlikely to see a major breakthrough.

The National Plan to Address Alzheimer's Disease

In May of 2012 the U.S. Department of Health and Human Services (HHS) released its first National Plan to Address Alzheimer's Disease. Using "Alzheimer's disease" as an umbrella term for all dementias, the Plan includes five main goals:

1) Prevent and effectively treat Alzheimer's disease by 2025;
2) Optimize care quality and efficiency;
3) Expand supports for people with Alzheimer's disease and their families;
4) Enhance public awareness and engagement; and
5) Track progress and drive improvement.

Although it's a lengthy and complex plan, its main elements look promising. For example, the Plan supports the education of health care providers about services available for people with Alzheimer's disease and their caregivers, so that patients and their families receive "counseling, support, or information about next steps." HHS will work with the Centers for Medicare and Medicaid Services to promote smoother transitions between care settings. The Plan champions more support for people with dementia who face unique challenges, such as racial and ethnic minorities, people with Down's syndrome (who almost always develop Alzheimer's disease as they age), and people with early-onset Alzheimer's disease. Offices for the Aging throughout the country will be encouraged to learn more about how caregivers can be connected with support services such as respite. And HHS will conduct a national survey to figure out why so many middle-aged people do not plan for long-term care.

I can see that one element of the National Plan falls short, however. While it calls for more training in dementia care for professionals such as physicians, nurses, social workers, and aides, it does not specify how many hours of training are ideal. I'm sure that both my mother and I would have felt less stress over the past seven years if every health care provider and professional caregiver we encountered had received at least a minimum number of hours of training in the specifics of dementia care. Currently, individual states may or may not require dementia education, and their regulations vary by industry (home care, adult day care, assisted living, nursing homes, hospitals, and hospice). Some states, for example, require absolutely no dementia education for staff in the dementia units of assisted living. The National Council of Certified Dementia Practitioners recommends a national standard of a minimum of 12 hours of initial dementia education for all health care professionals and front line staff in every industry, and then ongoing dementia education throughout the year. They also recommend that HHS study existing state regulations, and if HHS were to find that some states require more than 12 hours of training for dementia education, NCCDP recommends that federal regulations be developed to match the highest level of training.

Pending Legislation

HOPE

The Health Outcomes, Planning, and Education (HOPE) for Alzheimer's Act, in both the Senate and the House of Representatives, would increase early diagnosis, and improve access to information, care and support. According to the Alzheimer's Association, "Although Alzheimer's disease is diagnosed correctly up to 90 percent of the time by physicians with specialized training, as many as half of individuals meeting specific diagnostics for dementia never receive a diagnosis—and some evidence suggests it could be as high as 80 percent. The absence of a formal diagnosis of Alzheimer's deprives individuals of treatments and services that could help people and families facing Alzheimer's by improving symptoms, prolonging independence, and reducing caregiver stress. A formal and documented diagnosis opens access to valuable supports and services." The HOPE Act would also provide care planning visits with primary care physicians to discuss medical and community support services: "These valuable services help individuals with the disease and their caregivers better manage medications, engage in financial planning, and assess driving and safety issues in advance." These are exactly the kinds of issues (minus, perhaps, the medication coordination) that my mother needed help with years ago. If Dr. Gavin had been encouraged by federal legislation to have had these discussions with my mother on a regular basis, perhaps Mom would have given him permission to talk to me about these issues before she could no longer live alone, and I could have helped her that much earlier.

THE BREAKTHROUGH ACT

A second pending piece of legislation, the Breakthrough Act—reintroduced into the House of Representatives in 2011—called for "a federal commitment to Alzheimer's disease research to advance breakthrough treatments for people living with Alzheimer's disease." When I compared the original text of the 2009 version of the Act to the 2011 version, I found it discouraging that while the 2009 version called explicitly for an increase in Alzheimer's research funding in the NIH to $2 billion (from the current $450 million), the 2011 version has back-pedaled, omitting any specific request for an increase in funds. According to the 2011 Act, "The medical and research communities have the ideas, the technology, and the will, but need the Federal Government to commit to an innovative research approach, to find breakthroughs that will provide significant returns on investment and will save millions of lives."

Unfortunately, this version includes no dollar amount to support an "innovative research approach." It requires only that the NIH come up with budget estimates to carry out each of its recommended actions, "without regard to the probability that such amounts...will be appropriated."

In October 2011, the Alzheimer's Foundation of America published a bold report extolling the United States to catch up with the seven countries that already have national plans in place for Alzheimer's research, treatment, and support services, and to significantly increase our research funding. AFA played a large role in the passage of NAPA, and members serve on the new federal Advisory Council on Alzheimer's Research, Care, and Services.

The AFA also supports an increase in funding for the Cures Accelerations Network at the NIH, which would help reduce the delay—now an average of fourteen years—between the research of drugs and treatments and Food and Drug Administration approval. They recommend a substantial increase in funding not just for a cure for Alzheimer's disease, but for clinical research on earlier diagnosis and prevention, "safety issues; non-pharmacological behavioral interventions; end-of-life care; and support and dementia care training for family caregivers of all ages and ethnic backgrounds, clinicians—including primary care physicians, and direct care employees."

All of these research topics would have benefited both my mother and myself.

In October, masses of people in Canberra, Australia, took to the streets and marched on their capital, demanding more support for Alzheimer's research. In November, the Alzheimer's Association published a summary of the concerns of over 43,000 Americans affected by the disease. As part of the National Alzheimer's Project Act, 132 public input sessions over four months gathered comments and pleas from people across the country—people living with Alzheimer's, caregivers, researchers, health care providers, elder care professionals, community leaders, and others.

In his introduction to this report, Harry Johns, President and CEO of the Alzheimer's Association, writes, "We need a transformational plan. We need it urgently. It's time to roll up our sleeves and get it done."

I couldn't agree more.

Resources

For further information and support. These are some of my favorite books on dementia and caregiving, reports on dementia research and public policy, and organizations and Web sites supporting caregivers, but it is by no means an exhaustive list. For an annotated list of resources, please visit the Web site for this book, www.insidedementia.com.

BOOKS

Basting, Anne Davis. *Forget Memory: Creating Better Lives for People with Dementia.* Baltimore, MD: The Johns Hopkins University Press, 2009.

Bell, Virginia, and David Troxel. *The Best Friends Approach to Alzheimer's Care.* Baltimore, MD: Health Professions Press, 2003.

Berman, Claire. *Caring for Yourself While Caring for Your Aging Parents: How to Help, How to Survive.* New York: Owl Books, 2005.

Borrie, Cathie. *The Long Hello: The Other Side of Alzheimer's.* Vancouver, B.C.: Nightwing Press, 2010.

Boss, Pauline, Ph.D. *Loving Someone Who Has Dementia: How to Find Hope While Coping with Stress and Grief.* San Francisco, CA: Jossey-Bass, 2011.

Bryden, Christine. *Dancing with Dementia: My Story of Living Positively with Dementia.* Philadelphia: Jessica Kingsley Publishers, 2005.

Caposella, Cappy, and Sheila Warnock. *Share the Care: How to Organize a Group to Care for Someone Who Is Seriously Ill.* New York: Fireside, 2004.

Cohen, Elizabeth. *The House on Beartown Road: A Memoir of Learning and Forgetting.* New York: Random House, 2003.

Coste, Joanne Koenig. *Learning to Speak Alzheimer's: A Groundbreaking Approach for Everyone Dealing with the Disease.* New York: First Mariner Books, 2003.

DeBaggio, Thomas. *Losing My Mind: An Intimate Look at Life with Alzheimer's.* New York: The Free Press, 2002.

Geist, Mary Ellen. *Measure of the Heart: A Father's Alzheimer's, a Daughter's Return.* New York: Springboard Press, 2008.

Genova, Lisa. *Still Alice.* New York: Pocket Books, 2009.

Gillies, Andrea. *Keeper: One House, Three Generations, and a Journey into Alzheimer's.* New York: Broadway Paperbacks, 2009.

Gleckman, Howard. *Caring for Our Parents: Inspiring Stories of Families Seeking New Solutions to America's Most Urgent Health Crisis.* New York: St. Martin's Press, 2009.

Goldman, Connie. *The Gifts of Caregiving: Stories of Hardship, Hope and Healing*. Minneapolis, MN: Fairview Press, 2002.

Greenblat, Cathy Stein. *Alive with Alzheimer's*. Chicago: The University of Chicago Press, 2004.

———. *Love, Loss and Laughter: Seeing Alzheimer's Differently*. Guilford, CT: Lyons Press, 2012.

Gross, Jane. *A Bittersweet Season: Caring for Our Aging Parents—and Ourselves*. New York: Alfred A. Knopf, 2011.

Hadas, Rachel. *Strange Relation: A Memoir of Marriage, Dementia, and Poetry*. Philadelphia, PA: Paul Dry Books, 2011.

Jacobs, Barry J., Psy.D. *The Emotional Survival Guide for Caregivers—Looking After Yourself and Your Family While Helping an Aging Parent*. New York: Guilford Press, 2006.

Kane, Robert L., MD. *The Good Caregiver: A One-of-a-Kind Compassionate Resource for Anyone Caring for an Aging Loved One*. New York: Penguin Group, 2011.

Kane, Robert L., MD, and Joan C. West. *It Shouldn't Be This Way: The Failure of Long-Term Care*. Nashville, TN: Vanderbilt University Press, 2005.

Keith, Cindy. *Love, Laughter and Mayhem: Caregiver Survival Manual for Living with A Person with Dementia*. Port Charlotte, FL: BookLocker, 2010.

Kessler, Lauren. *Dancing with Rose: Finding Life in the Land of Alzheimer's*. New York: Penguin Group, 2007.

Kind, Viki. *The Caregiver's Path to Compassionate Decision-Making: Making Choices for Those Who Can't*. Austin, TX: Greenleaf Book Group, 2010.

LaPlante, Alice. *Turn of Mind*. New York: Atlantic Monthly Press, 2011.

Levine, Judith. *Do You Remember Me? A Father, a Daughter, and a Search for the Self*. New York: Free Press, 2004.

Lokvig, Jytte. *Alzheimer's A to Z: Secrets of Successful Caregiving*. Santa Fe, NM: Endless Circle Press, 2003.

Lokvig, Jytte, and John Becker. *Alzheimer's A to Z: A Quick-Reference Guide*. Oakland, CA: New Harbinger Publications, 2004.

Loverde, Joy. *The Complete Eldercare Planner, Revised and Updated Edition: Where to Start, Which Questions to Ask, and How to Find Help*. New York: Three Rivers Press, 2009.

Mace, Nancy L., and Peter V. Rabins. *The 36-Hour Day: A Family Guide to Caring for Persons with Alzheimer Disease, Related Dementing Illnesses, and Memory Loss in Later Life*. New York: Warner Books, 2006.

Marriott, Hugh. *The Selfish Pig's Guide to Caring: How to Cope with the Emotional and Practical Aspects of Caring for Someone*. London: Piatkus, 2003.

McCullough, Dennis. *My Mother, Your Mother: Embracing "Slow Medicine," the Compassionate Approach to Caring for Your Aging Loved Ones*. New York: HarperCollins, 2008.

McGowin, Diana Friel. *Living in the Labyrinth: A Personal Journey Through the Maze of Alzheimer's*. New York: Dell Publishing, 1994.

Miller, Sue. *The Story of My Father: A Memoir.* New York: Random House, 2003.

Mintz, Suzanne Geffen. *A Family Caregiver Speaks Up: It Doesn't Have to Be This Hard.* Herndon, VA: Capital Books, 2007.

Power, G. Allen. *Dementia Beyond Drugs: Changing the Culture of Care.* Baltimore, MD: Health Professions Press, 2010.

Radin, Lisa, and Gary Radin, eds. *What If It's Not Alzheimer's? A Caregiver's Guide to Dementia.* Amherst, NY: Prometheus Books, 2008.

Rubinstein, Nataly. *Alzheimer's Disease and Other Dementias: The Caregiver's Complete Survival Guide.* Minneapolis, MN: Two Harbors Press, 2011.

Sheehy, Gail. *Passages in Caregiving: Turning Chaos into Confidence.* New York: William Morrow, 2010.

Shulman, Alix Kates. *To Love What Is: A Marriage Transformed.* New York: Farrar, Straus and Giroux, 2008.

Simard, Joyce. *The End-of-Life Namaste Care Program for People with Dementia.* Baltimore, MD: Health Professions Press, 2007.

Span, Paula. *When the Time Comes: Families with Aging Parents Share Their Struggles and Solutions.* New York: Springboard Press, 2009.

Taylor, Richard. *Alzheimer's from the Inside Out.* Baltimore, MD: Health Professions Press, 2007.

Thomas, William H. *Life Worth Living: How Someone You Love Can Still Enjoy Life in a Nursing Home: The Eden Alternative in Action.* St. Louis, MO: Vanderwyk & Burnham, 1996.

———. *What Are Old People For?: How Elders Will Save the World.* St. Louis, MO: Vanderwyk & Burnham, 2007.

Thorndike, John. *The Last of His Mind: A Year in the Shadow of Alzheimer's.* Athens, OH: Swallow Press, 2009.

Whitman, Lucy, ed. *Telling Tales About Dementia: Experiences of Caring.* London: Jessica Kingsley Publishers, 2009.

Zeisel, John. *I'm Still Here: A Breakthrough Approach to Understanding Someone Living with Alzheimer's.* New York: Penguin Group, 2009.

RESEARCH REPORTS and POLICY RECOMMENDATIONS

AARP Public Policy Institute. *Valuing the Invaluable: 2011 Update: The Growing Contributions and Costs of Family Caregiving*, http://assets.aarp.org/rgcenter/ppi/ltc/i51-caregiving.pdf.

Alzheimer's Association. *Alzheimer's from the Frontlines: Challenges a National Alzheimer's Plan Must Address.* November, 2011, www.alz.org/documents_custom/napareport.pdf.

———. *2012 Alzheimer's Disease Facts and Figures.* http://www.alz.org/downloads/Facts_Figures_2012.pdf.

Alzheimer's Foundation of America. *No Time to Waste: Recommendations for an Integrated National Plan to Overcome Alzheimer's Disease.* October 2011. http://aspe.hhs.gov/daltcp/napa/cmtach17.pdf.

U.S. Department of Health and Human Services, *"National Plan to Address Alzheimer's Disease,"* May 15, 2012, http://aspe.hhs.gov/daltcp/napa/NatlPlan.pdf.

Working Mother Research Institute, *Women and Alzheimer's Disease: The Caregiver's Crisis,* June 2012, http://www.wmmsurveys.com/ALZ_report.pdf.

ORGANIZATIONS and WEB SITES

211 Information and Referral Search
www.211.org

Alzheimer's Association
www.alz.org phone: 800-272-3900

Caregiving.com
www.caregiving.com phone: 773-343-6341

Caring.com
www.caring.com

Caring From a Distance
www.cfad.org phone: 202-895-9465

Centers for Medicare and Medicaid Services
www.cms.gov

Children of Aging Parents
www.caps4caregivers.org

The Eden Alternative®
www.edenalt.org phone: 585-461-3951

Eden at Home®
www.edenalt.org/eden-at-home phone: 585-461-3951

Eldercare Locator
www.eldercare.gov phone: 800-677-1116

Engaging Alzheimer's
www.engagingalzheimers.com phone: 914- 844-6254

Family Caregiver Alliance
www.caregiver.org phone: 800-445-8106

The Green House Project®
http://thegreenhouseproject.org phone: 703-647-2311

Lotsa Helping Hands
www.lotsahelpinghands.com

Meals on Wheels
www.mowaa.org phone: 703-548-5558

National Academy of Elder Law Attorneys
www.naela.org phone: 703-942-5711

National Adult Day Services Association
www.nadsa.org phone: 877-745-1440

National Alliance for Caregiving
www.caregiving.org

National Association of Area Agencies on Aging
www.n4a.org phone: 202-872-0888

National Association of Professional Geriatric Care Managers
www.caremanager.org phone: 520-881-8008

National Board for Certified Counselors
www.nbcc.org phone: 336-547-0607

National Center for Assisted Living
www.ncal.org phone: 202-842-4444

National Center on Senior Transportation
http://seniortransportation.easterseals.com phone: 866-528-NCST

National Council of Certified Dementia Practitioners
www.nccdp.org phone (toll-free): 877-729-5191

National Family Caregivers Association
www.nfcacares.org phone: 301-942-6430

National Hospice and Palliative Care Organization
www.nhpco.org phone: 703-837-1500

Notes

EPIGRAPH

Christine Bryden, *Dancing with Dementia: My Story of Living Positively with Dementia* (Philadelphia: Jessica Kingsley Publishers, 2005), 150.

PREFACE

1 **One in eight people:** Alzheimer's Association, "2012 Alzheimer's Disease Facts and Figures," *Alzheimer's & Dementia*, Volume 8, Issue 2, p. 14. http://www.alz.org/downloads/facts_figures_2012.pdf. © 2012 Alzheimer's Association. All rights reserved.

1 **In the United States in 2011:** Alzheimer's Association, "2012 Alzheimer's Disease Facts and Figures," p. 31.

2 **In the United States in 2012:** Ibid., p. 51.

2 **William Thies, Ph.D., the Alzheimer's**: Alzheimer's Association, "International Survey Reveals Attitudes Towards Alzheimer's Diagnosis and Treatment," *Alzheimer's Association Finger Lakes Region Newsletter*, Fall 2011, 2, http://www.alz.org/rochesterny/documents/ALZ_Fall 011News3.pdf. © 2012 Alzheimer's Association. All rights reserved.

A NEW BEGINNING

17 **The Alzheimer's Association describes:** Alzheimer's Association, "Seven Stages of Alzheimer's," 2011, http://www.alz.org/alzheimers_disease_stages_of_alzheimers.asp. © 2012 Alzheimer's Association. All rights reserved.

20 **In May of 2011 an international**: Lab Tests Online, "Biomarkers Incorporated into Alzheimer's Disease Diagnostic Criteria," July 5, 2011, http://labtestsonline.org/news/biomarkers-incorporated-into-alzheimer-s-disease-diagnostic-criteria/.

OUR HISTORY

51 **The weight crept back on**: Kathleen Doheny, "Belly Fat in Midlife, Dementia Later? Study Shows Getting a Big Belly in Midlife Ups Risk of Dementia Later in Life," WebMD Health News, March 26, 2008, http://www.webmd.com/alzheimers/news/20080326/belly-fat-in-midlife-dementia-later.

51 **I will learn later that weight loss**: University of South Florida Health, "Unexplained Late-life Weight Loss May Be Early Predictor Of Alzheimer's Disease," ScienceDaily, Jun. 11, 2007, http://www.sciencedaily.com/releases/2007/06/070611092048.htm.

52 **Although this habit may have been:** The Murray Alzheimer Research and Education Program, University of Waterloo, "Tips and Strategies: An Inspirational Guide for People Like Us with Early-Stage Memory Loss," 2008, http://marep.uwaterloo.ca/products/BUFU/93711_tips.strategies.pdf.

SMALL INDIGNITIES

83 **According to Forbes.com:** Dan Ackman, "Retirement Doomsday," Forbes.com, May 4, 2005, http://www.forbes.com/2005/05/04/cx_da_0504topnews.html.

ALONE IN A CROWD

105 **I read in the *New York Times:*** Kolata, "Old but Not Frail: A Matter of Heart and Head," *New York Times*, October 5, 2006, sec. A.

LIVING GRIEF

186 **I leaf through a magazine:** Lauren Kessler, "The Life in There: years after her mother died of Alzheimer's, Lauren Kessler was still terrified of the disease. And so she decided to meet her fear head-on—by taking an entry-level job at an Alzheimer's facility. First came the shock. Then, amazingly, the awe. What she learned will change the way you think about the diagnosis we all dread." *O, The Oprah Magazine*, June 2007: 187+.

RECKONING

211 **In 2007 in New York State**: Community Health Advocates, "Section 5A: Medicaid in NY," June 2007, http://www.communityhealthadvocates.org/advocates-guide/medicaid-managed-care/medicaid-in-new-york#howspenddownworks.

211 **In 2011 the national average:** MetLife Mature Market Institute, "Market Survey of Long-Term Care Costs: The 2011 MetLife Market Survey of Nursing Home, Assisted Living, Adult Day Services, and Home Care Costs," October 2011, 7-9, http://www.metlife.com/assets/cao/mmi/publications/studies/2011/mmi-market-survey-nursing-home-assisted-living-adult-day-services-costs.pdf

SHARP AND SWEET

221 **Her departure reminds me again**: Lauren Kessler, *Dancing with Rose: Finding Life in the Land of Alzheimer's* (New York: Viking Penguin, 2007), 256.

FINANCIAL DISASTER

225 **She will soon qualify for Medicaid**: Evelyn Frank Legal Resources Program of Selfhelp Community Services, Inc., "Medicaid Spend-Down," New York Health Access, June 1, 2009, http://wnylc.com/health/entry/46/.

WHAT IF'S

229 **A few weeks later I read**: Jane E. Brody, "Putting Muscle Behind End-of-Life Issues," *New York Times*, Feb. 23, 2009, D7.

HONESTY

238 **In her book *Forget Memory***: Anne Davis Basting, *Forget Memory: Creating Better Lives for People with Dementia* (Baltimore: The Johns Hopkins University Press, 2009), 28. Reprinted with permission of The Johns Hopkins University Press.

239 **In *Learning to Speak Alzheimer's***: Joanne Koenig Coste, *Learning to Speak Alzheimer's: A Groundbreaking Approach for Everyone Dealing with the Disease* (New York: First Mariner Books, 2004), 77.

239 **John Zeisel writes in his book:** John Zeisel, *I'm Still Here: A Breakthrough Approach to Understanding Someone Living with Alzheimer's* (New York: Avery Trade, 2009), 157-8.

ANOTHER SEARCH FOR HOME

244 **Its fundamental tenet is that**: William H. Thomas, M.D., *Life Worth Living: How Someone You Love Can Still Enjoy Life in a Nursing Home* (Acton, MA: VanderWyk & Burnham, 1996), 7-23. Reprinted with permission of VanderWyk & Burnham, an imprint of Quick Publishing, LC, 888-PUBLISH, fax 314-993-4485, email quickpublishing@sbcglobal.net.

246 **According to Dr. Thomas, its founder:** Thomas, quoted in Camille Peri, "Talking with Bill Thomas: Reimagining Nursing Homes: The doctor who wants to revolutionize nursing homes talks about why old age should be a time of growth, not decline, and how we can make that happen," Caring.com, July 18, 2008, http://www.caring.com/interviews/interview-with-bill-thomas-about-pulling-the-plug-on-nursing-homes. ©Copyright 2008-2012, Caring.com. All Rights Reserved.

246 **Their website explains that**: THE GREEN HOUSE® Project, "Learn About Us," http://thegreenhouseproject.org/about-us/.

247 **To change the culture of elder care**: NCB Capital Impact, "THE GREEN HOUSE® Frequently Asked Questions," http://www.ncbcapitalimpact.org/defaultaspx?id=508#GHculturechange.

247 **According to the blogstream Changing Aging**: Kavan Peterson, "The Green House Project Featured in USA Today, Plus New Consumer Toolkit," ChangingAging Blogstream, April 1, 2011, http://changingaging.org/blog/2011/04/01/the-green-house-project-featured-in-usa-today-plus-new-consumer-toolkit/.

247 **Instead of working all day**: St. John's Home, "THE GREEN HOUSE® Project: St. John's Green House® Project: Transforming Elder Services in New York," 2011, http://www.stjohnshome.com/green-house-project.

247 **According to the Green House Project**: THE GREEN HOUSE® Project, "Consumer Tool Kit," 16.

248 **With the financial support**: THE GREEN HOUSE® Project, "RWJF Announce $10 Million Expand Green House Access to Low-Income Elders," Sept. 8, 2011, http://thegreenhouseproject.com/rwjf-announce-10-million-expand-green-house-access-to-low-income-elders/.

248 **By September 2011 there will be**: THE GREEN HOUSE® Project, "Evaluating THE GREEN HOUSE® Model," p.1, http://thegreenhouseproject.org/wp-content/uploads/2011/10/green_house_research-1-pager-with-map_September-2011.pdf.

248 **According to the developer of one**: St. John's Home.

248 **Care can be paid for by**: THE GREEN HOUSE® Project, "Consumer Tool Kit," p.3, http://thegreenhouseproject.org/wp-content/uploads/2011/04/The-Green-House-Project_Consumer-Toolkit_rev3.pdf.

248 **An average of fifty percent**: Kavan Peterson, "Live Grow Thrive: Green House Model Promotes Growth," ChangingAging Blogstream, Jan. 11, 2011, http://changingaging.org/blog/2011/0111/live-grow-thrive-green-house-model-promotes-growth/.

248 **The AARP calls the project**: THE GREEN HOUSE® Project, "RWJF Announce $10 Million Expand Green House Access to Low-Income Elders."

249 **In his book *What Are Old People For?***: William H. Thomas, M.D., *What Are Old People For? How Elders Will Save the World* (Acton, MA: VanderWyk & Burnham, 2004), 234-235.

249 **Doctors, social workers, and physical**: Peterson, "Live Grow Thrive."

FOUR KINDS OF PAIN

254 **I learn later that when**: Jean Carper, *100 Simple Things You Can Do to Prevent Alzheimer's and Age-Related Memory Loss* (New York: Little, Brown and Company, 2010), 26-28.

REBOUND

256 **In Barbara Ehrenreich's book *Bright-Sided***: Barbara Ehrenreich, *Bright-Sided: How the Relentless Promotion of Positive Thinking Has Undermined America* (New York: Metropolitan Books, 2009), 9-44.

SMALL PLEASURES

264 **Dr. G. Allen Power, author**: G. Allen Power, M.D., Plenary Presentation. "Dementia Beyond Drugs: Changing the Culture of Care," *Ithaca College Gerontology Institute 2010 Annual Conference: Dignity, Compassion, and Choice: New Approaches to Geriatric Care*, Campus Center, Ithaca College, Ithaca, New York, Sept. 30, 2010.

IS IT ALZHEIMER'S, OR NOT?

274 **According to the collection of essays**: John. Q. Trojanowski, M.D., Ph.D., Foreword, in *What If It's Not Alzheimer's?: A Caregiver's Guide to Dementia*, Lisa Radin and Gary Radin, eds. (Amherst, New York: Prometheus Books, 2008), 15.

275 **In one of the essays in**: Murray Grossman, "What Is Frontotemporal Dementia? A Clinical Perspective," in Radin and Radin, 46.

276 **As Katherine P. Rankin points**: Katherine P. Rankin, "Altered Relationships: Adapting to Emotions and Behavior," in Radin and Radin, 219.

276 **On the other hand, when I read**: Rachel Hadas, *Strange Relation: A Memoir of Marriage, Dementia, and Poetry* (Philadelphia: Paul Dry Books, 2011), xi,119.

AFTERWORD

283 **Indeed, I'd follow the advice of**: Nataly Rubinstein, *Alzheimer's Disease and Other Dementias: The Caregiver's Complete Survival Guide* (Minneapolis, MN: Two Harbors Press, 2011), 56-63.

APPENDIX A: IS THERE A TEST TO DIAGNOSE ALZHEIMER'S DISEASE?

289 **According to Dr. Frank Longo**: Frank Longo, MD, PhD, "The Coming Epidemic of Dementia and How It Can Be Diagnosed, Treated, and Prevented," Stanford School of Medicine, Stanford, CA, address, May 2012, http://scopeblog.stanford.edu/2012/05/31/stanford-neuroscientist-discusses-the-coming-dementia-epidemic/.

290 **The Alzheimer's Association reserves**: "Alzheimer's Association Statement on Florbetapir PET Amyloid Imaging," Alzheimer News, Jan. 21, 2011, http://www.alz.org/news_and_events_pet_amyloid_imaging.asp ©2012 Alzheimer's Association, all rights reserved.

290 **A spinal fluid test has been**: Jenny Marder, "Spinal Fluid Test a New Tool for Diagnosing Alzheimer's Disease," *PBS Newshour*, August 10, 2010, http://www.pbs.org/newshour/rundown/2010/08/doctors-may-be-able-to.html.

290 **Many doctors and researchers**: Gina Kolata, "In Spinal Fluid Test, an Early Warning on Alzheimer's," *New York Times*, August 8, 2010, http://www.nytimes.com/2010/08/10/health/research/10spinal.html.

290 **In May of 2011, an international**: Lab Tests Online, "Biomarkers Incorporated into Alzheimer's Disease Diagnostic Criteria," July 5, 2011, http://labtestsonline.org/news/biomarkers-incorporated-into-alzheimer-s-disease-diagnostic-criteria/.

291 **That's a tall order**: Alzheimer's Association, "Frequently Asked Questions: Publication of New Criteria and Guidelines for Alzheimer's Disease Diagnosis," April 2011, 1-3, http://www.alz.org/documents_custom/Alz_Diag_Criteria_FAQ.pdf. ©2012 Alzheimer's Association, all rights reserved.

291 **Dr. Jack Diamond, the scientific**: Jack Diamond, M.D., quoted in Nick Krewen, "Alzheimer's Cases Predicted to Rise 1000 Percent: What's Being Done to Find a Cure," www.samaritanmag.com, October 12, 2011. http://samaritanmag.com/859/alzheimers-cases-predicted-rise-1000-percent-whats-being-done-find-cure.

292 **The international workgroup**: Lab Tests Online, "Biomarkers Incorporated into Alzheimer's Disease Diagnostic Criteria," July 5, 2011, http://labtestsonline.org/news/biomarkers-incorporated-into-alzheimer-s-disease-diagnostic-criteria/.

292 **As Diamond points out**: Diamond, quoted in Krewen.

APPENDIX B: MEDICATIONS APPROVED TO RELIEVE SYMPTOMS OF ALZHEIMER'S DISEASE

293 **Two types of prescription medications:** National Institutes of Health, National Institute on Aging, "Alzheimer's Disease Medications Fact Sheet," April 9, 2012, http://www.nia.nih.gov/alzheimers/publication/alzheimers-disease-medications-fact-sheet.

293 **They include Aricept:** Dementia SOS: Colorado's Dementia News and Resource Center, "The Medications for Alzheimer's," Jan. 17, 2012, http://www.coloradodementia.org/tag/razadyne.

293 **A two-and-a-half-year:** Alireza Atir, MD, PhD; Lynn W. Shaughnessy, BS; Joseph J. Locasio, PhD; John H. Growdon, MD, "Long-term Course and Effectiveness of Combination Therapy in Alzheimer Disease," *Alzheimer's Disease and Related Disorders,* 22(3): 209-211, July/September 2008, http://www.ncbi.nlm.nih.gov/pmc/articles/PMC2718545/

294 **A study published in the *Journal:*** Pierre N. Tariot, MD; Martin R. Farlow, MD; George T. Grossberg, MD; Stephen M. Graham, PhD; Scott McDonald, PhD; Ivan Gergel, MD; for the Memantine Study Group, "Memantine Treatment in Patients with Moderate to Severe Alzheimer Disease Already Receiving Donepezil," *Journal of the American Medical Association,* 2004; 291(3): 317-324. www.jamanetwork.com/article.aspx?articleid=198033.

APPENDIX C: RISK FACTORS AND ANTIDOTES FOR DEMENTIA

295 **As a large French multi-center**: Gillette, et al., "Prevention of Progression to Dementia in the Elderly: Rationale and Proposal for a Health-Promoting Memory Consultation (Task Force Members)," *The Journal of Nutrition, Health and Aging*, Oct. 12, 2008, http://iana-congress.eu/docs/sophie.pdf, 6.

295 **A 2011 study published**: G.L. Bowman, ND, MPH, L.C., Silbert, MD, MCR, D. Howieson, PhD, H.H. Dodge, PhD, M.G. Traber, PhD, B. Frei, PhD, J.A. Kaye, MD, J. Shannon, PhD, MPH, and J.F. Quinn, MD, "Nutrient Biomarker Patterns, Cognitive Function, and MRI Measures of Brain Aging," *Neurology*, December 28, 2011, http://www.neurology.org/content/early/2011/12/28/WNL.0b013e3182436598.abstract.

295 **Because aerobic exercise increases:** Alzheimer's Association, "Stay Physically Active," http://www.alz.org/we_can_help_stay_physically_active.asp. Copyright © 2012 Alzheimer's Association®. All rights reserved.

296 **A recent study by neurologists:** Aron S. Buchman, MD, Patricia Boyle, PhD, Li Yu, PhD, Raj C. Shah, MD, Robert S. Wilson, PhD, and David A. Bennett, MD, "Total Daily Physical Activity and the Risk of AD and Cognitive Decline in Older Adults," ScienceDaily, April 18, 2012, www.sciencedaily.com/releases/2012/04/120418203530.htm.

296 **In another study, subjects who walked:** Longo, "The Coming Epidemic of Dementia and How It Can Be Diagnosed, Treated, and Prevented."

296 **In a third study, people with mild cognitive:** Ibid.

297 **The Alzheimer's Association recommends:** Alzheimer's Association, "Adopt a Brain-Healthy Diet," http://www.alz.org/we_can_help_adopt_a_brain_healthy_diet.asp. Copyright © 2012 Alzheimer's Association®. All rights reserved.

298 **In a study of elderly people:** Guyonnet S Gillette, G. Abellan Van Kan, S. Andrieu, J.P. Aquino, C. Arbus, J.P. Becq, C. Berr, S. Bismuth, B. Chamontin, T. Dantoine, J.F. Dartigues, B. Dubois, B. Fraysse, T. Hergueta, H. Hanaire, C. Jeandel, S. Lagleyre, F. Lala, F. Nourhashemi, P.J. Ousset, F. Portet, P. Ritz, P. Robert, Y. Rolland, C. Sanz, M. Soto, J. Touchon, and B. Vellas, cited in Mary A. Rogers and Kenneth M. Langa, "Untreated Poor Vision: A Contributing Factor to Late-Life Dementia," *American Journal of Epidemiology*, Oxford University Press, Vol.171, no.6, Feb. 11, 2010, http://aje.oxfordjournals.org/content/171/6/728.full#fn-group-1.

299 **A study led by the University:** Jennifer O'Brien, "Sleep Apnea Linked to Increased Risk of Dementia in Elderly Women," The University of California, San Francisco, Aug. 9, 2009, http://www.ucsf.edu/news/2011/08/10408/sleep-apnea-linked-increased-risk-dementia-elderly-women.

299 **Other researchers find:** Michael C. Purdy, "Marker for Alzheimer's Disease Rises During Day, Falls with Sleep: Up-and-down cycle flattens as age disrupts pattern," Sept. 26, 2011, Washington University in St. Louis, http://news.wustl.edu/news/Pages/22709.aspx.

299 **In 2010, researchers in Milan:** American Academy of Sleep Medicine, "CPAP Therapy Restores Brain Tissue in Adults with Sleep Apnea, Study Finds," ScienceDaily, June 7, 2010, http://www.sciencedaily.com/releases/2010/06/100607065550.htm.

300 **We know that the obese:** American Thoracic Society, "Relationship Between Overnight Rostral Fluid Shift and Obstructive Sleep Apnea in Non-obese Men," ajrccm.atsjournals.org, Nov. 14, 2008, http://ajrccm.atsjournals.org/cgi/content/abstract/179/3/241.

300 **The National Sleep Foundation:** National Sleep Foundation, "Sleep Apnea and Sleep," http://www.sleepfoundation.org/article/sleep-related-problems/obstructive-sleep-apnea-and-sleep.

300 **According to the American Sleep:** American Sleep Apnea Association, "Sleep Apnea," http://www.sleepapnea.org/learn/sleep-apnea.html.

301 **Vaccines to reduce the build-up:** Alzheimer Society of Canada, "Alzheimer's Disease and Related Dementias—In Pursuit of a Cure."

301 **Similar trials in 2000 resulted:** Diamond, quoted in Krewen.

301 **Other studies are being conducted:** Alzheimer Society of Canada, "Alzheimer's Disease and Related Dementias—In Pursuit of a Cure."

301 **Startling new research in February:** Gina Kolata, "Path is Found for the Spread of Alzheimer's," *New York Times*, Feb. 1, 2012, http://www.nytimes.com/2012/02/02/health/research/alzheimers-spreads-like-a-virus-in-the-brain-studies-find.html.

APPENDIX D: IS IT "ALL IN THE FAMILY"?

303 **In Alzheimer's disease over age sixty:** Alzheimer's Disease Education & Referral (ADEAR) Center, A Service of the National Institute on Aging, National Institutes of Health, U.S. Department of Health and Human Services, "Alzheimer's Disease Genetics Fact Sheet," NIH Publication No. 11-6424, June 2011, http://www.nia.nih.gov/Alzheimers/Publications/geneticsfs.htm.

APPENDIX F: SWEET POISON: THE TOXIC TIDE OF SUGAR

305 **After I discovered that:** "Sleep Apnea May Increase Insulin Resistance," American Thoracic Society press release, May 17, 2010, http://www.thoracic.org/media/press-releases/conference/articles/2010/ih-and-insulin-resistance.pdf, 1.

305 **During sleep, insulin levels:** Denise Grady, "Link Between Diabetes and Alzheimer's Deepens," *New York Times*, July 17, 2006, http://www.nytimes.com/2006/07/17/health/17alzheimer.html.

305 **Also, a study at the University:** "Sleep Apnea May Increase Insulin Resistance."

305 **Many researchers now describe:** "Discovery Supports Theory of Alzheimer's Disease as Form of Diabetes," Northwestern University press release, http://www.research.northwestern.edu/news/stories/2008/klein.html.

306 **Someone like me who is:** Grady.

306 **Being overweight or obese:** W.L. Xu, M.D., Ph.D., A.R. Atti, M.D., Ph.D., M. Gatz, Ph.D., N.L. Pederson, Ph.D., B. Johansson, Ph.D., and L. Fratiglioni, M.D., Ph.D., "Abstract: Midlife Overweight and Obesity Increase Late-Life Dementia Risk: A Population-Based Twin Study," *Neurology*, May 3, 2011, http://www.neurology.org/content/76/18/1568.abstract.

306 **In 2010, researchers at Kyushu:** Fisher Center, "Diabetes Linked to Brain Damage of Alzheimer's Disease."

306 **Another study has determined:** Kolata, "A Squirt of Insulin May Delay Alzheimer's," *New York Times*, Sept. 13, 2011, D5.

306 **Some anti-diabetic drugs, such as:** Alzheimer Society of Canada, "Alzheimer's Disease and Related Dementias–In Pursuit of a Cure," http://www.alzheimer.ca/english/media/research2011.htm.

306 **A team at Northwestern University:** Northwestern University press release.

307 **In fact, a product called Axona®**: "Genetic Profile Identified for Alzheimer's Patients Showing Heightened Response to Accera's Breakthrough Product Axona®," Accera, Inc. news release, Freshnews.com, Oct. 17, 2011, http://www.freshnews.com/news/562352/genetic-profile-identified-alzheimer-s-patients-showing-heightened-response-accera-s-br.

307 **A prescription, FDA-designated**: Accera, Inc., "Axona," http://www.accerapharma.com/axona.html.

308 **I follow the advice of Gary**: Gary Taubes, *Good Calories, Bad Calories: Fats, Carbs, and the Controversial Science of Diet and Health* (New York: Anchor Books, 2008), 454.

308 **Although I don't pay attention**: Emily Deans, M.D., "The Case for Evolution—Octopuses, Grandmothers, Iceland, and Poor Dr. T. Colin Campbell," Evolutionary Psychiatry (blog), Sept. 4, 2010, http://evolutionarypsychiatry.blogspot.com/2010/09/case-for-evolution-octopi-grandmothers.html.

309 **Referring to the connection between**: Deans, "Examining the Complicated Factors That Predispose Us to Dementia," Evolutionary Psychiatry (blog), Sept. 20, 2011, http://www.psychologytoday.com/blog/evolutionary-psychiatry/201109/alzheimers-and-high-blood-sugar.

APPENDIX G: THE BENEFITS OF "MEMORY CONSULTATIONS" AND EARLY DIAGNOSIS

310 **A French multi-center task force**: Gillette, et al., 6.

310 **Memory care programs in**: University of Rochester Medical Center, "Comprehensive Memory Care Program Fills Vital Need," 2011, http://www.urmc.rochester.edu/referring-physicians/urmc-connection/spring-2010/facilities-and-programs/dementia-clinic.cfm.

311 **According to the Centers for Medicare**: Charles Fiegel, "Medicare's Missed Checkups: Few Seniors Get Wellness Exam," American Medical Association, May 2, 2011, http://www.ama-assn.org/amednews/2011/05/02/gvsa0502.htm.

311 **Many doctors—including my mother's**: Alzheimer's Association, "International Survey Reveals Attitudes Towards Alzheimer's Diagnosis and Treatment," Alzheimer's Association International Conference press release, Paris, July 20, 2011, http://alz.org/aaic/wednesday_1230amCT_news_release_intl_ survey.asp.

312 **In their 2011 report *Alzheimer's Disease:*** Alzheimer's Association, "2011 Alzheimer's Disease Facts and Figures," 47, http://www.alz.org/downloads/Facts_Figures_2011.pdf. ©2012 Alzheimer's Association, all rights reserved.

APPENDIX H: PLANNING FOR LONG-TERM CARE

313 **In March of 2010**: Paula Span, "The New Old Age: Behind the Class Act, a Numbers Game," *New York Times*, Sept. 18, 2011, http://newoldage.blogs.nytimes.com/2011/10/18/behind-the-class-act-a-numbers-game/

313 **By the fall of 2011, though**: Gardiner Harris and Robert Pear, "Still No Relief in Sight for Long-Term Needs," *New York Times*, Oct. 25, 2011, Sec. D, 1,6.

314 **If CLASS had existed successfully**: Paula Span, "The New Old Age: Details on the Class Act," *New York Times*, April 29, 2010, http://newoldage.blogs.nytimes.com/2010/04/29/details-on-the-class-act/.

314 **This amount would have been**: Long Term Care Partners, "The Federal Long Term Care Insurance Program: Frequently Asked Questions," http://www.ltcfeds.com/help/faq/basics.html.

314 **According to the Family Caregiver**: Family Caregiver Alliance, "What Is Long-Term Care?" http://www.caregiver.org/caregiver/jsp/content_node.jsp?nodeid=440.

315 **If CLASS had existed years ago:** The Henry J. Kaiser Foundation, "Health Care Reform and the CLASS Act," April 2012, 2, http://www.kff.org/healthreform/upload/8069.pdf.

315 **According to Howard Gleckman**: Howard Gleckman, *Caring for Our Parents: Inspiring Stories of Families Seeking New Solutions to America's Most Urgent Health Crisis* (New York: St. Martin's Press, 2009), 177.

316 **The average annual premium**: American Health Care Association, National Center for Assisted Living, "Financial Information: Understanding Long Term Care Insurance," 3, http://www.longtermcareliving.com/pdf/ltc_insurance.pdf.

316 **Private long-term care insurance**: Gleckman, 34-246.

APPENDIX I: LONG-TERM CARE AN INTENTIONAL COMMUNITY

318 **He says that "people will only**: Charles Durrett, *Senior Cohousing: A Community Approach to Independent Living* (Berkeley: McCamant/Durett, 2005), 123,184.

319 **Durrett describes how some**: Ibid., 123-24.

APPENDIX J: CONFRONTING THE EPIDEMIC AT THE NATIONAL LEVEL AND BEYOND

320 **According to the Alzheimer's Association**: Alzheimer's Association press release, "Alzheimer's Breakthrough Act: Alzheimer's Association Statement," Washington, D.C., July 23, 2009, http://www.alz.org/national/documents/statements_breakthroughact.pdf.

320 **In their May 2011 report**: Susan Peschin, *Penny Wise, Pound Foolish: Fairness and Funding at the National Institute on Aging*, Alzheimer's Foundation of America, May 2011, http://www.alzfdn.org/documents/NIA%20Report-Final.pdf, 3-4.

320 **The AFA quotes Sam Gandy**: Sam Gandy, M.D., Ph.D., quoted in Alzheimer's Foundation of America, *Penny Wise, Pound Foolish*, 9.

321 **The National Plan to Address:** U.S. Department of Health and Human Services, National Plan to Address Alzheimer's Disease, May 15, 2012, http://aspe.hhs.gov/daltcp/napa/NatlPlan.pdf.

322 **Currently, individual states may:** Stimson, Sandra, CALA ADC AC-BC CDP CDCM, Founder and Executive Director, National Council of Certified Dementia Practitioners, personal communication, June 19, 2012.

323 **According to the Alzheimer's Association**: Alzheimer's Association, "The Hope for Alzheimer's Act," 2010, http://www.kintera.org/site/pp.asp?c=mmKXLbP8E&b=6301189. ©2012 Alzheimer's Association, all rights reserved.

324 **A second pending piece of legislation**: Congress, House, Alzheimer's Breakthrough Act of 2011, 112th Congress, 1st sess., HR 1897, May 13, 2011, 1, http://www.kintera.org/atf/cf/%7BB96E2E84-AF7D-4656-9C86-285306F00E19%7D/HR%201897%20%28GPO%205-30%29.pdf.

324 **When I compared the original text**: Govtrack.us, "Text of S. 1492 [111th]: Alzheimer's Breakthrough Act of 2009," http://www.govtrack.us/congress/billtext.xpd?bill=s111-1492.

324 **the 2011 version has back-pedaled**: Congress, House, Alzheimer's Breakthrough Act of 2011, 8.

325 **The AFA also supports**: Alzheimer's Foundation of America, *No Time to Waste: Recommendations for an Integrated National Plan to Overcome Alzheimer's Disease*, Oct. 2011, 8-9, http://aspe.hhs.gov/daltcp/napa/cmtach17.pdf.

325 **In his introduction to this report**: Harry Johns, Introduction, *Alzheimer's from the Frontlines: Challenges a National Alzheimer's Plan Must Address*, Alzheimer's Association, 2011, 3. ©2012 Alzheimer's Association, all rights reserved.

Acknowledgments

This is my favorite part—thanking the many people who've cheered me on. Without their support I doubt I could have worked on this project for seven years.

Since I have changed the names and descriptions of most of the people and places in this book, I cannot use full names here for the people who live in my city. I wish I could. If you are one of those local folks, forgive me.

Laura Shaine Cunningham, the Artistic Director of the Memoir Institute, helped me shape the manuscript into the book it is today, and I cannot thank her enough. Every new author should be as lucky as I was to meet Laura at the Omega Institute's Memoir Festival and to build the kind of working relationship that we enjoy. I will be forever grateful for her insight, editing skills and unwavering support of this project.

Kathryn Craft, the owner of Writing-Partner.com, read an early draft in 2008 and wrote a brilliant, twelve-page evaluation of the manuscript. I also want to thank Jerry Waxler of the Memory Writers Network, for teleclasses he offered through the National Association of Memoir Writers on the craft of writing memoir, and for his thoughtful evaluation and editing of an early draft. Kathryn and Jerry's suggestions guided me through my first major revision of the manuscript. In 2012 Kathryn read the manuscript again, and I am indebted to her for her clear thinking and incisive edits.

When I took Professor Katy G.'s class "The Art of the Personal Essay" back in 2005 as an employee of a local university, she encouraged me to turn my writing on caregiving into the chapters of a book. Without her early faith in me I may never have considered the idea. I thank her for this early encouragement, and for reading and commenting on two drafts.

Many thanks to Meg D., Carol H., Rachael S., Aileen F., Laura B. and Linda V. for reading an early version and offering suggestions, and to Meg. D., Joyce C., Suzanne K., Sara K., and Laura B. for reading and commenting on a later draft. Many thanks also to Judy E. for applying her stellar proofreading skills to the final draft.

Thank you to Lucy Whitman, Marc Wortmann, Viki Kind, Sandra Stimson, Cindy Keith, Sharon K. Brothers, Nataly Rubinstein, and Joyce Simard for reviewing the advance copy and offering their suggestions.

Through their work as life coaches, Meg D. and Jaya helped me to stay motivated to sit my bottom in a chair each day and write, even when the goal of a finished book seemed absolutely impossible.

Another professional editor, Mickey P., evaluated an early draft, and I want to thank her for pointing out its flaws; over time I was able to appreciate her directness, and, I hope, to make the necessary revisions.

Over several years I wrote many scenes in this book sitting at Ellen S.'s dining room table in her weekly writing group. I will always appreciate her gentle comments and editing suggestions, and her ongoing support. I also thank Irene Z. and her women's writing group for providing another safe place to explore my feelings about caregiving and my family history.

Barbara V., my boss for several years during the course of this story, always believed in "family first" and allowed me to take time off to attend to my mother's medical emergencies. Barbara also supported my request to work from home to give me more time to write. A former community college president, and an English major as an undergraduate, she believed in the importance of using writing to "bear witness" to injustice and suffering; social change, she would say, often begins with story.

Lee R., a coworker who lost her own mother to Alzheimer's disease, has always been generous with her empathy and emotional support.

Susan Daffron and James Byrd of Logical Expressions, who have self-published twelve books, have guided me through the publishing process. I also thank the other members of their Author's Circle for their inspiration and practical suggestions.

Wayne G., a neighbor and fellow writer, promised several years ago to always ask me how my book was going. He followed through, year after year, always with an encouraging smile.

Many thanks to all of Mom's "angels" who have brightened her days—the staff in her facilities, plus Laura G., Suzanne K. and Terry M.

My mother, Judy, has always been my most steadfast cheerleader. She told me years ago that she felt certain that I would end up writing a book of some sort. If she happened to be in it, she said, she asked only that I be "kind" to my "old Mom." I hope that I've honored her wish.

I thank my family—my dear husband Ben, son Andrew and daughter Morgan—for their patience with my new job of writing. I especially thank Morgan, who, at age 10, told me early on in the project that a book about taking care of Grammy was a good idea because "it will help other people in your situation know that they are not alone."

Index

INDEX

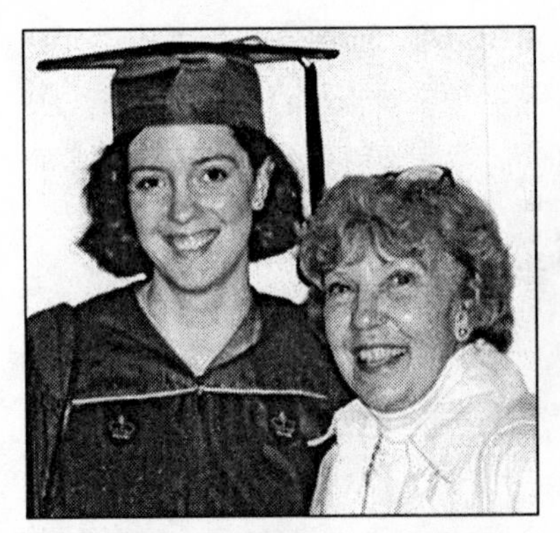

Mom at 62, and me at 30, in 1995

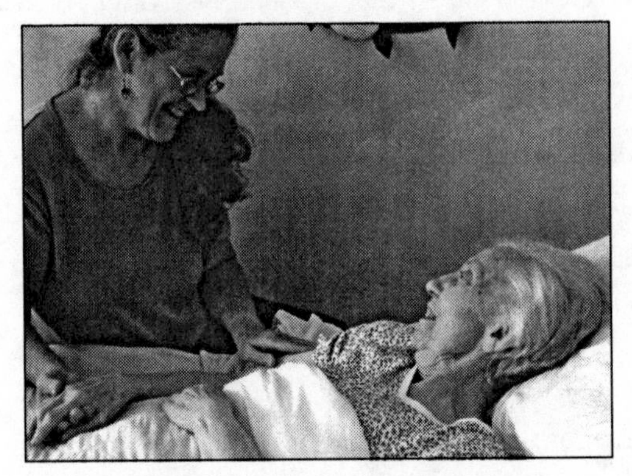

Mom, 77, with Suzanne, a massage therapist who specializes in bodywork for elders, in 2010

(photo by Jason Kates van Staveren)

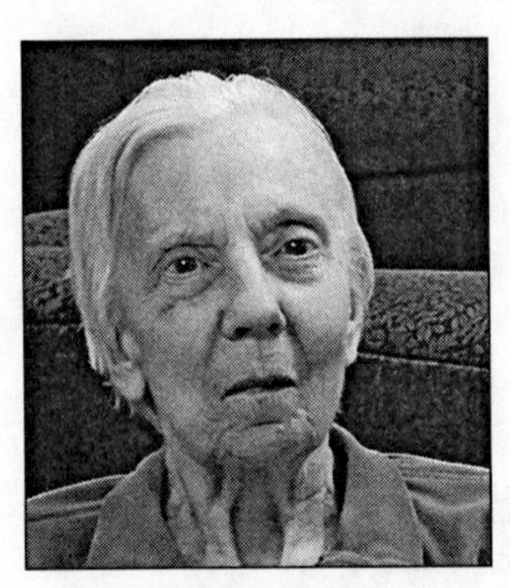

Mom, 79, in 2012